Pharmacological Therapies for Peripheral Vascular Disease

PHARMACOLOGICAL THERAPIES FOR PERIPHERAL VASCULAR DISEASE

Edited by

Debabrata Mukherjee MD FACC
Tyler Gill Professor of Interventional Cardiology
Director of Peripheral Intervention Program
Gill Heart Institute
Division of Cardiovascular Medicine
University of Kentucky
Lexington, KY
USA

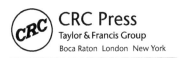

CRC Press
Taylor & Francis Group
Boca Raton London New York

CRC Press is an imprint of the
Taylor & Francis Group, an **informa** business

CRC Press
Taylor & Francis Group
6000 Broken Sound Parkway NW, Suite 300
Boca Raton, FL 33487-2742

First issued in paperback 2019

© 2005 by Taylor & Francis Group, LLC
CRC Press is an imprint of Taylor & Francis Group, an Informa business

No claim to original U.S. Government works

ISBN-13: 978-1-84184-457-2 (hbk)
ISBN-13: 978-0-367-39262-8 (pbk)

A CIP record for this book is available from the British Library.

Visit the Taylor & Francis Web site at
http://www.taylorandfrancis.com

and the CRC Press Web site at
http://www.crcpress.com

CONTENTS

LIST OF CONTRIBUTORS

Dinesh Arab MD
Loyola University Medical Center
Maywood, IL
USA

Herbert D Aronow MD MPH
Assistant Professor of Medicine
Director, Cardiac Catheterization Laboratory
Philadelphia Veteran's Affairs Medical Center
University & Woodland Avenues
Philadelphia, PA
USA
and
Director, Peripheral Intervention
Hospital of the University of Pennsylvania
Cardiovascular Division
Philadelphia, PA
USA

John R Bartholomew MD
Department of Cardiovascular Medicine
Section of Vascular Medicine
Cleveland Clinic Foundation
Cleveland, OH
USA

Deepak L Bhatt MD FACC FSCAI FESC
Director, Interventional Cardiology
    Fellowship
Staff, Cardiac, Peripheral, and Carotid
    Intervention
Cleveland Clinic Foundation
Department of Cardiovascular Medicine
Cleveland, OH
USA

Stanley J Chetcuti MD FACC
Clinical Assistant Professor, Division of
    Cardiology
University of Michigan Health System
University Hospital
Ann Arbor, MI
USA

Leslie Cho MD
Assistant Professor of Medicine
Loyola University Medical Center
Stritch School of Medicine
Maywood, IL
USA

Eron D Crouch MD
Division of Cardiology (Fellow)
University of North Carolina
Chapel Hill, NC
USA

Rupal Dumasia MD
Division of Cardiology
University of Michigan Health System
University Hospital
Ann Arbor, MI
USA

Kim A Eagle MD
Albion Walter Hewlett Professor of Internal
    Medicine
Division of Cardiology
University of Michigan Cardiovascular Center
Ann Arbor, MI
USA

Douglas Joseph DO
Section of Vascular Medicine
Cleveland Clinic Foundation
Cleveland, OH
USA

Samir R Kapadia MD
Department of Cardiovascular Medicine,
Staff, Interventional Cardiology
Peripheral Vascular Intervention
Cleveland Clinic Foundation
Cleveland, OH
USA

Juhana Karha MD
Department of Cardiovascular Medicine,
Cleveland Clinic Foundation
Cleveland, OH
USA

Victor M Mejia MD
Hospital of the University of Pennsylvania
Cardiovascular Medicine Division-9022 E.
 Gates
Philadelphia, PA
USA

Debabrata Mukherjee MD FACC
Tyler Gill Professor of Interventional
 Cardiology
Associate Professor of Internal Medicine
Director of Peripheral Intervention
 Program
Associate Director for Cardiac
 Catheterization Laboratories
Gill Heart Institute, Division of
 Cardiovascular Medicine
University of Kentucky
Lexington, KY
USA

David S Lee MD
Department of Cardiovascular Medicine
Cleveland Clinic Foundation
Cleveland, OH
USA

John Pfeifer MD
Professor of Vascular Surgery
Director, Division of Ambulatory Venous
 Surgery
University of Michigan School of Medicine
Ann Arbor, MI
USA

Bertram Pitt MD
Associate Chair, Internal Medicine
 Department
Professor, Internal Medicine Department
Int MED-Cardiology
Ann Arbor, MI
USA

Sanjay Rajagopalan MD
Associate Professor
Mount Sinai School of Medicine
New York, NY
USA

Joel Reginelli MD
Cardiology Center of Cincinnati
Cincinnato, OH
USA

Marco Roffi MD
Andreas Grüntzig Cardiovascular
 Catheterization Laboratories
Cardiology
University Hospital
Zurich
Switzerland

Steven R Steinhubl MD
Director of Cardiovascular Education and
 Clinical Research
Associate Professor of Medicine
Division of Cardiology
University of Kentucky
Lexington, KY
USA

PREFACE

Peripheral arterial disease is the most common manifestation of atherosclerosis and is associated with a three- to five-fold increased risk of cardiovascular mortality compared to age-matched controls. Several recent studies have demonstrated that atherosclerotic risk factors are very prevalent in patients with peripheral arterial diseases; but these patients are treated less intensively with lipid-lowering agents, antiplatelet therapy or antihypertensives. Although there are numerous texts focusing on vascular interventions, there is no comprehensive text that discusses optimal medical therapy of patients with peripheral arterial diseases. Vascular interventionalists have an opportunity not only to provide high quality and appropriate vascular interventions, but also to seize the peri-procedural moment in aggressively treating the underlying atherosclerotic process through lifestyle modifications and effective pharmacological therapies. Ultimately, attention to these disease management opportunities is more likely to affect both quality and quantity of life than the procedures themselves.

Pharmacological Therapies for Peripheral Vascular Disease is the first text that comprehensively discusses optimal pharmacotherapy for patients with peripheral arterial and venous disorders. This text discusses optimal use of anti-platelet agents, lipid-lowering agents, statins, angiotensin converting enzyme inhibitors and other adjunctive pharmacological therapies for patients with peripheral arterial diseases. Several recent studies have documented the underutilization of these therapies and have demonstrated significantly better outcomes when these agents are used appropriately. A separate section on venous diseases discusses contemporary management of deep venous thrombosis and pulmonary embolism, including the role of newer antithrombotic agents and also discusses the use of compression stockings and sclerosing agents for treatment of varicose veins.

Debabrata Mukherjee
April 2005

ARTERIAL DISEASES

1. LIFESTYLE CHANGES AND RISK FACTOR MODIFICATION

Debabrata Mukherjee

Atherosclerosis is the most common cause of peripheral arterial disease (PAD). PAD is a common medical problem and affects a large segment of the adult population, with an age-adjusted prevalence of 12–20%.[1–3] Available data suggest that approximately 50% of patients with PAD are asymptomatic, 45% have intermittent claudication, and only a small minority presents with symptoms of ischemic pain at rest, ulceration, or gangrene.[4] In regards to natural history studies, patients with PAD have a threefold to fivefold increased risk of cardiovascular mortality compared to age-matched controls.[5] Overall mortality rate increases with the severity of vascular disease, which is most commonly assessed by the ankle–brachial index (ABI)[6–9] or with increasing symptom severity.[10]

Natural history

The natural history regarding limb loss in most patients with PAD is fairly benign except in diabetics and smokers. Symptoms of claudication remain stable or improve with time in 65–70% of patients due to development of collateral vessels and <25% ever need surgery or angioplasty.[4,11] There is a low risk of losing a limb – only 1.4% per year progress to critical life-threatening ischemia; however, patients with diabetes and smokers have an increased overall amputation risk. Most of the morbidity and mortality is related to cardiovascular and cerebrovascular events in individuals with PAD and average life span is shortened by 10 years depending on the status of the cardiovascular system.[3] The worst prognosis is in diabetic patients who smoke.

Cardiovascular and cerebrovascular assessment

Symptomatic peripheral vascular disease carries at least a 30% risk of death within 5 years and almost 50% within 10 years, primarily due to myocardial infarction (60%) or stroke (12%).[12,13] Even asymptomatic individuals with peripheral vascular diseases (ABI <0.9) have a twofold to fivefold increased risk of fatal or nonfatal cardiovascular events.[12] Because cardiovascular events are the most

3

common adverse outcome in patients with peripheral vascular disease, the physician should perform some assessment in estimating the patient's risk for coronary artery disease. The physician should certainly take into account both the presence of conventional and non-conventional risk factors, including blood pressure, family history, lipid profile, smoking history, diabetes, and homocysteine levels. Should there be a high index of suspicion for the presence of coronary artery disease, a functional study may be indicated to document any reversible coronary ischemia. Patients with symptomatic intermittent claudication and clinical suspicion of carotid atherosclerosis should be assessed for cerebral vascular disease by referring the patient for a duplex ultrasound of the carotid arteries. It is important to recall that only 40% of patients with significant internal carotid artery stenosis will actually have an audible cervical bruit.[14] Therefore, patients that have symptomatic PAD may be screened for significant carotid artery disease with a carotid artery duplex examination if clinically indicated.

Lifestyle changes

Lifestyle changes are extremely important in addressing/modifying the risk factors for PAD. Exercise, better nutrition, and weight loss all reduce future cardiovascular risk. The issues of weight loss, optimal nutrition, exercise, and smoking cessation are long-term goals that call for patient-specific discussions. Despite being a powerful risk factor for PAD, cigarette smoking remains one of the most difficult factors to modify (i.e. getting patients to quit).

A regular walking regimen is extremely helpful. The best program is a stop–start walking regimen and includes regular daily walks, 30–45 min/day, at least 3 times/week, for at least 6 months. Individuals should walk as far as possible using near-maximal pain as a signal to stop and resume walking when pain goes away. A typical supervised exercise program is 60 min in duration and is monitored by a skilled nurse or technician. Patients should be encouraged to walk primarily on a treadmill, since this most closely reproduces walking in the community setting. The initial workload of the treadmill is set to a speed and grade that bring on claudication pain within 3–5 min. Patients walk at this work rate until they achieve claudication of moderate severity. They then rest until the claudication abates, and then resume exercise. This repeated on-and-off form of exercise is continued throughout the supervised rehabilitation setting. On a weekly basis, patients should be reassessed clinically as they are able to walk further and further at their chosen workload. This then will necessitate an increase in speed or grade or both to allow patients to successfully work at harder and harder workloads. This scenario will then induce a training benefit.[15] Patients can walk 180–400% farther with this regimen. There is some evidence that older age, femoropopliteal disease, and more aggressive exercise sessions predict better response to treatment.[16] Exercise training, therefore, is an effective treatment for claudication, the primary symptom of peripheral arterial disease. The benefit of exercise may be related to several mechanisms, including measurable improvements in endothelial vasodilator function, skeletal muscle metabolism, blood viscosity, and inflammatory responses.[17]

The progression of peripheral vascular atherosclerosis is significantly greater in patients who continue to smoke. The incidence of myocardial infarction 10 years after the diagnosis of claudication was 11% in former smokers and 53% in active smokers and 10-year overall survival rates were 82% in former smokers and 42% in active smokers, respectively.[18] Complete cessation of tobacco use should be the goal in these patients. Stopping smoking can reduce the 5-year amputation risk tenfold and decrease the mortality rate by 50%.[19–22] Referral to a smoking cessation program and the use of nicotine patches or gum are recommended and may be helpful. Bupropion, an anxiolytic agent, has been effective when added to brief regular counseling sessions in helping patients to quit smoking. Family members who live in the same household should be encouraged to quit smoking to help reinforce the patient's effort and to decrease the risk of secondhand smoke for everyone.

Risk factor modification

The risk factors for PAD are similar to those for coronary and cerebrovascular disease (Box 1.1). The higher the blood pressure, the greater is the risk of claudication. In the Framingham study, the relative risk of claudication was 1.27 if the systolic blood pressure was 20 mmHg higher than normal and 1.62 if it was 40 mmHg higher.[23] Thus, it is imperative to adequately control blood pressure. Strict control of hypertension results in a slowdown of disease progression and a reduction in cardiovascular events.[24] Optimal blood pressure control is an important goal, and hypertensive patients should be appropriately educated. Systolic and diastolic blood pressures should be in the normal range (systolic less than 135 mmHg, diastolic less than 85 mmHg).

Box 1.1 Risk factors for peripheral arterial disease

- Hypertension
- Dyslipidemia
  - o High low-density lipoprotein (LDL)
  - o High triglycerides
  - o Low high-density lipoprotein (HDL)
- Diabetes mellitus
- Smoking
- Sedentary lifestyle

Hypercholesterolemia doubles the incidence of intermittent claudication, and is found in as many as 50% of patients with PAD.[25] Angiographic studies have confirmed that lipid lowering retards the progression of femoral atherosclerosis[26,27] and HMG CoA reductase inhibitors have been shown to reverse the progression of carotid atherosclerosis.[28,29] All patients should be on lipid-lowering therapy with a target LDL of <100 mg/dL (refer to Chapter 4).

Diabetes mellitus and PAD is an ominous combination, because of the rapid progression to ischemic rest pain and ulceration in these patients.[30] Among the risk factors for amputation in diabetic patients, neuropathic symptoms and lack of outpatient diabetes education are predictors[31] and should be integrated in the evaluation of PAD. Optimal glycemic control should be a consideration in these individuals. Persons with claudication and diabetes have an overall amputation risk of 20% and a 5-year mortality rate of up to 50%. Tight glucose control (HbA1c <7.0%) in diabetics has been shown to lower acute and 1-year mortality rates and microvascular disease.[32] The UK Prospective Diabetes Study (UKPDS) demonstrated that the control of glycemia reduces diabetes-related events, including heart attacks (16% reduction, $p = 0.052$), for newly detected type 2 diabetics.[33-35] Overweight patients should be recommended a structured weight-loss program, with emphasis on the importance of regular exercise and a lifelong prudent diet to maintain ideal weight.

Future directions

A new drug that might counteract obesity and smoking at the same time was reported at the annual scientific sessions of the American College of Cardiology in 2004.[36] Preliminary data on the effects of rimonabant on obesity and smoking coincided with a study by the Centers for Disease Control (CDC) on smoking, soon being overtaken by obesity as the nation's number one underlying death factor. Rimonabant is the first of a new class of drugs that block the cannabinoid receptor 1 (CB1). The CB1 receptor is thought to play an important role in certain aspects of human behavior and metabolism – specifically, it is thought to play a role in obesity, smoking habits, and lipid and glucose metabolism. The STRATUS-US (STudies with Rimonabant And Tobacco USe), a double-blind, placebo-controlled study, showed that rimonabant doubled the odds of quitting smoking compared to placebo ($p = 0.002$). Among patients completing the study, prolonged abstinence was significantly higher in the patients treated with 20 mg of rimonabant (36.2%) when compared with patients treated with placebo (20.6%). Results of a Phase III clinical trial (RIO-Lipids or Rimonabant In Obesity), comparing rimonabant to placebo, found that overweight or obese patients with untreated dyslipidemia (high triglycerides, low HDL-cholesterol) lost almost 20 lbs

(8.6 kg) when treated for a year with rimonabant 20 mg. Weight loss was accompanied by a decrease in waist size of 3.4 inches (9.1 cm), demonstrating a significant reduction in abdominal obesity, an independent marker for heart disease. Dramatic improvements were also seen in lipid profile with a 23% increase in HDL-cholesterol (good cholesterol) and a 15% decrease in triglycerides. Improvements in glucose tolerance and insulin levels were also observed. In another important finding, the number of patients diagnosed at baseline with metabolic syndrome who were treated with rimonabant 20 mg was reduced by half. If these results are validated in future studies, this agent could play an important role in preventing vascular diseases as an adjunct to lifestyle and risk factor modification.

Key points
- Atherosclerosis is the most common cause of peripheral arterial disease.
- The most common symptom of patients with peripheral arterial disease is intermittent claudication.
- Symptomatic peripheral vascular disease carries at least a 30% risk of death within 5 years and almost 50% within 10 years, primarily due to myocardial infarction (60%) or stroke (12%).
- Complete cessation of tobacco use should be the goal in patients with peripheral vascular disease.
- Lifestyle changes are extremely important in addressing/modifying the risk factors for PAD.
- Intensive risk factor modification is an important part of management of peripheral vascular disease.

References

1. Hiatt WR, Marshall JA, Baxter J, et al. Diagnostic methods for peripheral arterial disease in the San Luis Valley Diabetes Study. J Clin Epidemiol 1990;43:597–606.

2. Criqui MH, Fronek A, Barrett-Connor E, et al. The prevalence of peripheral arterial disease in a defined population. Circulation 1985;71:510–15.

3. Mukherjee D, Yadav JS. Update on peripheral vascular diseases: from smoking cessation to stenting. Cleve Clin J Med 2001;68:723–33.

4. McDaniel MD, Cronenwett JL. Basic data related to the natural history of intermittent claudication. Ann Vasc Surg 1989;3:273–7.

5. McKenna M, Wolfson S, Kuller L. The ratio of ankle and arm arterial pressure as an independent predictor of mortality. Atherosclerosis 1991;87:119–28.

6. Newman AB, Siscovick DS, Manolio TA, et al. Ankle-arm index as a marker of atherosclerosis in the Cardiovascular Health Study. Cardiovascular Heart Study (CHS) Collaborative Research Group. Circulation 1993;88:837–45.

7. Newman AB, Shemanski L, Manolio TA, et al. Ankle-arm index as a predictor of cardiovascular disease and mortality in the Cardiovascular Health Study. The Cardiovascular Health Study Group. Arterioscler Thromb Vasc Biol 1999;19:538–45.

8. Vogt MT, Cauley JA, Newman AB, Kuller LH, Hulley SB. Decreased ankle/arm blood pressure index and mortality in elderly women. JAMA 1993;270:465–9.

9. Vogt MT, McKenna M, Anderson SJ, Wolfson SK, Kuller LH. The relationship between ankle-arm index and mortality in older men and women. J Am Geriatr Soc 1993;41:523–30.

10. Criqui MH, Langer RD, Fronek A, et al. Mortality over a period of 10 years in patients with peripheral arterial disease. N Engl J Med 1992;326:381–6.

11. McAllister FF. The fate of patients with intermittent claudication managed nonoperatively. Am J Surg 1976;132:593–5.

12. Tierney S, Fennessy F, Hayes DB. ABC of arterial and vascular disease. Secondary prevention of peripheral vascular disease. BMJ 2000;320:1262–5.

13. Ouriel K. Peripheral arterial disease. Lancet 2001;358:1257–64.

14. Ziegler DK, Zileli T, Dick A, Sebaugh JL. Correlation of bruits over the carotid artery with angiographically demonstrated lesions. Neurology 1971;21:860–5.

15. Nehler MR, Hiatt WR. Exercise therapy for claudication. Ann Vasc Surg 1999;13:109–14.

16. Golledge J. Lower-limb arterial disease. Lancet 1997;350:1459–65.

17. Stewart KJ, Hiatt WR, Regensteiner JG, Hirsch AT. Exercise training for claudication. N Engl J Med 2002;347:1941–51.

18. Jonason T, Bergstrom R. Cessation of smoking in patients with intermittent claudication. Effects on the risk of peripheral vascular complications, myocardial infarction and mortality. Acta Med Scand 1987;221:253–60.

19. Krupski WC. The peripheral vascular consequences of smoking. Ann Vasc Surg 1991;5:291–304.

20. Dormandy J, Heeck L, Vig S. The natural history of claudication: risk to life and limb. Semin Vasc Surg 1999;12:123–37.

21. Dormandy J, Heeck L, Vig S. Predicting which patients will develop chronic critical leg ischemia. Semin Vasc Surg 1999;12:138–41.

22. Verhaeghe R. Epidemiology and prognosis of peripheral obliterative arteriopathy. Drugs 1998;56:1–10.

23. Stamler J, Stamler R, Neaton JD. Blood pressure, systolic and diastolic, and cardiovascular risks. US population data. Arch Intern Med 1993;153:598–615.

24. Mohler IE. Peripheral arterial disease. Curr Treat Options Cardiovasc Med 1999;1:27–34.

25. Kannel WB, Skinner JJ Jr, Schwartz MJ, Shurtleff D. Intermittent claudication. Incidence in the Framingham Study. Circulation 1970;41:875–83.

26. Walldius G, Erikson U, Olsson AG, et al. The effect of probucol on femoral atherosclerosis: the Probucol Quantitative Regression Swedish Trial (PQRST). Am J Cardiol 1994;74:875–83.

27. Blankenhorn DH, Azen SP, Crawford DW, et al. Effects of colestipol-niacin therapy on human femoral atherosclerosis. Circulation 1991;83:438–47.

28. Furberg CD, Adams HP Jr, Applegate WB, et al. Effect of lovastatin on early carotid atherosclerosis and cardiovascular events. Asymptomatic Carotid Artery Progression Study (ACAPS) Research Group. Circulation 1994;90:1679–87.

29. Mercuri M, Bond MG, Sirtori CR, et al. Pravastatin reduces carotid intima-media thickness progression in an asymptomatic hypercholesterolemic Mediterranean population: the Carotid Atherosclerosis Italian Ultrasound Study. Am J Med 1996;101:627–34.

30. Jonason T, Ringqvist I. Diabetes mellitus and intermittent claudication. Relation between peripheral vascular complications and location of the occlusive atherosclerosis in the legs. Acta Med Scand 1985;218:217–21.

31. Reiber GE, Pecoraro RE, Koepsell TD. Risk factors for amputation in patients with diabetes mellitus. A case-control study. Ann Intern Med 1992;117:97–105.

32. Malmberg K, Norhammar A, Wedel H, Ryden L. Glycometabolic state at admission: important risk marker of mortality in conventionally treated patients with diabetes mellitus and acute myocardial infarction: long-term results from the Diabetes and Insulin-Glucose Infusion in Acute Myocardial Infarction (DIGAMI) study. Circulation 1999;99:2626–32.

33. Intensive blood-glucose control with sulphonylureas or insulin compared with conventional treatment and risk of complications in patients with type 2 diabetes (UKPDS 33). UK Prospective Diabetes Study (UKPDS) Group. Lancet 1998;352:837–53.

34. Effect of intensive blood-glucose control with metformin on complications in overweight patients with type 2 diabetes (UKPDS 34). UK Prospective Diabetes Study (UKPDS) Group. Lancet 1998;352:854–65.

35. Tight blood pressure control and risk of macrovascular and microvascular complications in type 2 diabetes: UKPDS 38. UK Prospective Diabetes Study Group. BMJ 1998;317:703–13.

36. Effects of rimonabant in the reduction of major cardiovascular risk factors. Results from the STRATUS-US Trial (smoking cessation in smokers motivated to quit) and the RIO-LIPIDS Trial (weight reducing and metabolic effects in overweight/obese patients with dyslipidemia). American College of Cardiology Scientific Sessions, March 7–10, 2004, New Orleans.
http://www.acc04online.org/daily/news/newssummary.asp?sid=1&stid=14&newsld=2004-03-09

2. CILOSTAZOL AND PENTOXIFYLLINE IN THE TREATMENT OF PERIPHERAL ARTERIAL DISEASES

Dinesh Arab and Leslie Cho

Introduction

Patients with peripheral arterial disease (PAD) are at increased risk of death, when compared with age-matched healthy controls. Patients with PAD, whether symptomatic or not, are six times more likely to die within 10 years, when compared to patients without PAD.[1-4] This excess mortality is present even if coronary artery disease is not clinically present. McDermott et al[5] showed that risk factors in patients with peripheral vascular disease are less likely to be treated than in patients with coronary artery disease.

In addition, patients with PAD have decreased exercising capacity. This sets up a cycle of sedentary lifestyle that impacts the quality of life of patients and facilitates the progression of atherosclerosis. The improvement of symptoms without either a pharmacological or non-pharmacological intervention is unlikely, making appropriate therapy for PAD critical.[6] The treatment for PAD includes risk factor modification and therapy to prevent cardiovascular events, pharmacological therapy for claudication, exercise training for the treatment of claudication, and either surgical or endovascular revascularization.

Pharmacological therapy of claudication

The two drugs that are approved by the Food and Drug Administration (FDA) for claudication are pentoxifylline and cilostazol.

Pentoxifylline

Pentoxifylline is a methylxanthine derivative that improves blood flow by decreasing blood viscosity and improving red blood cell flexibility. This is thought to occur due to a reduction of plasma fibrinogen concentrations.[7,8] Limitation of blood flow may be due to a combination of obstructive atherosclerosis and hemorheological factors. Poiseuille's law, when applied to the circulatory system, describes an inverse relationship between blood flow and viscosity. Erythrocyte flexibility is one of the factors determining viscosity.[9,10] Patients with intermittent claudication have been shown to have a marked decrease in erythrocyte flexibility.[11,12] In addition, pentoxifylline inhibits membrane-bound phosphodiesterase, which in turn leads to an increase in cyclic monophosphate. This leads to inhibition of platelet aggregation, a decrease in thromboxane synthesis and an increase in prostacyclin synthesis. These effects lead to an increase in blood flow to the microvasculature, resulting in an increase in tissue perfusion.[13]

Pharmacokinetics

Pentoxifylline is absorbed orally and is approximately 45% bound to plasma proteins. Pentoxifylline is broken down to metabolites I and V, whose plasma concentrations are five and eight times greater than the parent compound. The pharmacokinetics of pentoxifylline and metabolite V (the major biotransformed product) is dose-related and nonlinear. The major method of excretion is primarily renal. The effects of hepatic and renal dysfunction on the pharmacokinetics of pentoxifylline have not been well studied.

Clinical efficacy

Pentoxifylline has been studied in the treatment of intermittent claudication, with conflicting results (Table 2.1, page 15). The main determinants assessed were symptomatic improvement in walking distance studies. These studies measured the initial claudication distance (ICD) and the absolute claudication distance (ACD). ICD is the amount of distance walked prior to the onset of claudication, whereas ACD is the total amount of distance covered until the patient stops walking. ICD is regarded as a more sensitive measure of treatment response, being less influenced by patient factors such as motivation and pain tolerance. Porter et al[14] assessed the safety and efficacy of pentoxifylline for intermittent claudication in a multicenter, double-blind, placebo-controlled, parallel group study involving 128 patients. The primary end point was an improvement in the ICD and the ACD. Pentoxifylline, given in doses from 600 mg/day to 1200 mg/day, resulted in an improvement in both mean ICD (179 m vs 158 m, $p = 0.016$), and mean ACD (247 vs 229 m, $p = 0.035$). The most common side effect with pentoxifylline was nausea.

Lingarde et al[15] conducted a double-blind study that compared pentoxifylline with placebo in 150 patients with moderately severe PAD. Patients were followed for a 6-month period. The end points were ICD and ACD. There was a statistically significant improvement in the ACD. Patients with PVD of greater than 1-year duration and patients with ankle–brachial index (ABI) of less than 0.8 improved more significantly when compared to placebo. Other studies have shown a similar increase in walking distance with the use of pentoxifylline.[16–18] In contrast, a study by Green et al[19] did not show any significant benefit of pentoxifylline on severity of symptoms or lifestyle changes in patients with intermittent claudication.

A meta-analysis of 12 studies in 612 patients[20] demonstrated that pentoxifylline improved pain-free walking distance and the ACD in patients with moderate intermittent claudication. Patients treated with pentoxifylline were able to walk, on average, 30 m more than control patients on a treadmill, which is equivalent to 90 m on flat ground. Due to the heterogeneity of the trials reviewed, the effect of pentoxifylline on various subgroups such as smokers, diabetics, and patients with hypertension could not be determined.

Cilostazol

Cilostazol is a quinolinone derivative that has been approved for the treatment of intermittent claudication since 1999 by the FDA. Cilostazol is a cyclic nucleotide phosphodiesterase (PDE) type 3 inhibitor. The PDEs act by affecting the intracellular concentration of cyclic adenosine monophosphate (cAMP) and cyclic guanosine monophosphate (cGMP). Cilostazol causes an increase in cAMP and cGMP, which affects the phosphorylation of protein kinase A substrates (Fig. 2.1). Cilastazol inhibits platelet aggregation, decreases vascular smooth muscle cell (VSMC) proliferation, causes VSMC relaxation and causes vasodilation.[21–25]

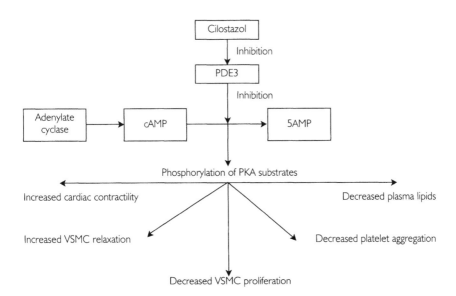

Figure 2.1 *Mechanism of action and effects of cilostazol. PDE3, phosphodiesterase type 3; PKA, cAMP-dependent protein kinase substrates; VSMC, vascular smooth muscle cells. (Adapted with permission from Liu et al. Cilastazol. Cardiovascular Drug Reviews 2001;19:369–86.)*

In addition cilostazol has a beneficial effect on lipid metabolism.[26] This includes a moderate reduction in triglycerides and an increase in high-density cholesterol (HDL). Cilostazol does not affect low-density cholesterol (LDL).

Pharmacokinetics

Cilostazol is well absorbed after oral administration and peaks in plasma about 3 hours after oral administration. Cilostazol is metabolized by the hepatic cytochrome P450 enzymes, particularly isoenzymes 3A4 and 2C19. Cilostazol and its metabolites have an elimination half-life of 12 hours and are predominantly excreted in urine. Drugs that affect the cytochrome P450 pathway can cause significant interactions with cilostazol. Drugs such as diltiazem, erythromycin, omeprazole, ketoconazole, and grape fruit juice, may increase cilostazol levels. Cilostazol is well tolerated with aspirin. Co-administration of a single dose of warfarin, while on a twice-daily dose of 100 mg cilostazol, did not alter the warfarin pharmacokinetics, prothrombin time or partial thromboplastin time. However, the effects of multiple doses of warfarin are unknown. Cilostazol can be given to patients with mild hepatic and renal impairment, without an adjustment in dosage. Cilostazol should be administered with caution in patients with moderate-to-severe hepatic impairment.[27–29]

PDE type 3 inhibitors cause an increase in cardiac contractility, and prototype drugs such as milrinone and enoximone have been used in the treatment of congestive heart failure (CHF). Milrinone and enoximone, when used in the treatment of CHF, have been associated with increased mortality, presumably due to their proarrhythmic action.[30,31] Due to a similar mode of action of cilostazol, the FDA has issued a black box warning, contraindicating the use of cilostazol in patients with CHF of any severity. Patients with significant CHF have been excluded in all the major trials involving cilostazol. The direct effect of cilostazol on mortality in CHF has not been studied. Other side effects of cilostazol include headache, diarrhea, and palpitations. These side effects rarely require discontinuation of the drug and respond to symptomatic treatment.

Clinical efficacy

Cilostazol was first approved in Japan for the treatment of PVD and critical leg ischemia. There have been four randomized, placebo-controlled trials of cilostazol in the United States (Table 2.2). Dawson et al[32] studied 81 patients, randomized in a 2:1 ratio, to either cilostazol or placebo. The study duration was 12 weeks, and the dose of cilostazol used was 100 mg twice a day. Primary end points were ICD and ACD. Secondary outcomes included ABI and safety. Treatment with cilostazol resulted in a 35% (p <0.01) increase in ICD and a 41% increase in ACD (p <0.01). There was no difference in resting

Table 2.1 Summary of major randomized trials using pentoxifylline for the treatment of intermittent claudication. Trials included had at least a 2-month follow-up

Study	N	Duration (months)	ICD (m)		p-value	ACD (m)		p-value
			Drug	Placebo		Drug	Placebo	
Porter et al[14]	128	6	179	158	0.016	247	229	0.035
Lindgarde et al[15]	150	6	139	126	NA	504	420	0.023
Roekaerts and Deleers[16]	36	6	1029	555	<0.05	1228	742	<0.05
Ernst et al[17]	40	3	364	384	NS	504	420	NA
Di Perri and Guerrini[18]	24	2	360	215	<0.05	NA	NA	NA
Gillings et al[21]	128	6	140	128	0.012	195	193	NS

ICD, initial claudication distance; ACD, absolute claudication distance; m, meters; NA, not studied; NS, not significant.

Table 2.2 Summary of trials using cilostazol for intermittent claudication

Study	N	Duration (months)	ICD (m)		p-value	ACD (m)		p-value
			Drug	Placebo		Drug	Placebo	
Dawson et al[32]	81	3	112	84	0.007	231	152	0.002
Money et al[33]	239	4	NA	NA	NA	332	281	<0.01
Beebe et al[34]	516	6	137.9	95.5	<0.01	258	174	<0.01
Dawson et al[35]	698	6	218	180	0.02	350	300	0.0002

ICD, initial claudication distance; ACD, absolute claudication distance; m, meters; NA, not studied; NS, not significant.

or post-exercise ABI. Money et al[33] studied the effects of cilostazol on walking distance in 239 patients with intermittent claudication. The study design was a randomized, double-blind, placebo-controlled, multicenter trial. The duration of the trial was 16 weeks. Patients treated with cilostazol showed an improvement over placebo in ACD at weeks 8, 12, and 16. The mean improvement in ACD at 16 weeks was 96.4 m (47%) in the cilostazol group and 31.4 m (12.9%) in the placebo group ($p < 0.001$). In addition, unlike the previous study, cilostazol treatment was associated with an improvement in ABI. The most frequent side effects were headache, diarrhea, and dizziness.

In a larger multicenter, randomized trial, Beebe et al[34] studied the effects of 516 patients with intermittent claudication. Patients were randomized to receive cilostazol 100 mg, 50 mg, or placebo twice a day, orally for 24 weeks. Outcome measures were ACD, ICD, quality of life, and all-cause mortality. Cilostazol treatment resulted in an improvement in symptoms at 4 weeks and the benefit was sustained at all time points. At 24 weeks, patients receiving 100 mg of cilostazol twice a day had a 51% increase in maximal walking distance ($p < 0.001$ vs placebo), whereas those who received cilostazol 50 mg twice a day, had a 38% improvement in maximal walking distance ($p < 0.001$ vs placebo). There was no difference between groups in the incidence of combined cardiovascular morbidity or all-cause mortality.

Dawson et al[35] compared the efficacy of cilostozol to pentoxifylline and placebo in a randomized, double-blind study involving 698 patients. The cilostazol-treated group had a mean increase in ACD of 107 m from baseline as compared to 64 m in the pentoxifylline group and 65 m in the placebo group. This change was statistically significant ($p < 0.001$), in favor of the cilostazol arm when compared to the other two groups. There was no difference between the pentoxifylline and placebo groups. There was a significant improvement ($p < 0.001$) in the ICD (94 m vs 74 m), between the cilostazol-treated groups and the pentoxifylline groups. The change in ICD between the pentoxifylline and placebo groups was not statistically significant. Death and serious side effects were similar in all groups.

Miscellaneous drugs (refer to Chapter 9)

Levocarnitine and propionyl levocarnitine have been studied for the treatment of intermittent claudication. These drugs are thought to act by improving the metabolism of skeletal muscle, thereby improving exercise performance. Propionyl levocarnitine has not been approved for use in the United States. Two small trials have shown that both pain-free and maximal treadmill walking distance were improved in patients treated with propionyl levocarnitine when compared to placebo. No definite recommendations can be made on these drugs in the absence of larger controlled trials. Other drugs used in the treatment of PVD include prostaglandins, naftidrofuryl, chelation, vitamin E and testosterone. These drugs are currently not recommended for the treatment of intermittent claudication or PVD as there are few data to support any benefit.

Key points

- Cilostazol is the drug of choice for the treatment of intermittent claudication.
- Pentoxifylline can be used as an alternative drug for the treatment of symptomatic claudication with limited efficacy.
- Cilostazol is contraindicated in patients with heart failure and left ventricular dysfunction.
- A number of agents such as L-arginine, prostaglandins and levocarnitine are currently being tested for the treatment of claudication.

References

1. Dormandy J, Heeck L, Vig S. Lower-extremity atherosclerosis as a reflection of a systemic process: implications for concomitant coronary and carotid disease. Semin Vasc Surg 1999;12:118–22.

2. Criqui MH, Langer RD, Fronek A, et al. Mortality over a period of 10 years in patients with peripheral arterial disease. N Engl J Med 1992;326:381–6.

3. Hertzer NR, Beven EG, Young JR, et al. Coronary artery disease in peripheral vascular patients. A classification of 1000 coronary angiograms and results of surgical management. Ann Surg 1984;199:223–33.

4. Aronow WS, Ahn C. Prevalence of coexistence of coronary artery disease, peripheral arterial disease, and atherothrombotic brain infarction in men and women >= 62 years of age. Am J Cardiol 1994;74:64–5.

5. McDermott MM, Mehta S, Ahn H, Greenland P. Atherosclerotic risk factors are less intensively treated in patients with peripheral arterial disease than in patients with coronary artery disease. J Gen Intern Med 1997;12:209–15.

6. McDermott MM, McCarthy W. Intermittent claudication: the natural history. Surg Clin North Am 1995;75:581–90.

7. Trental (pentoxifylline) product information. Kansas City, MO: Hoechst Marion Roussel; January 1998.

8. Ward A, Clissold SP. Pentoxifylline: a review of its pharmacodynamic and pharmacokinetic properties, and its therapeutic efficacy. Drugs 1987;34:50–97.

9. Reid HL, Dormandy JA, Barnes AJ, et al. Impaired red cell deformity in peripheral vascular disease. Lancet 1976;1:666.

10. Dormandy JA. Clinical importance of blood viscosity. Viscositas 1979;1:5.

11. Ehrly AM, Koehler HJ. Altered deformability of erythrocytes from patients with chronic occlusive arterial disease. Vasa 1976;319.

12. Dormandy JA, Hoare E, Colley J, et al. Clinical, hemodynamic, rheological, and biochemical findings in 126 patients with intermittent claudication. Br Med J 1973;4:576.

13. Ernst E. Pentoxifylline for intermittent claudication: a critical review. Angiology 1994;45:339–45.

14. Porter JM, Cutler BS, Lee BY, et al. Pentoxifylline efficacy in the treatment of intermittent claudication: multicenter controlled double-blind trial with objective assessment of chronic occlusive arterial disease patients. Am Heart J 1982;104:66–72.

15. Lindgarde F, Jelnes R, Bjorkman H, et al. Conservative drug treatment in patients with moderately severe chronic occlusive peripheral arterial disease. Scandinavian Study Group. Circulation 1989;80:1549–56

16. Roekaerts F, Deleers L. Trental 400 in the treatment of intermittent claudication: results of long-term, placebo-controlled administration. Angiology 1984;35:396–406.

17. Ernst E, Kollar L, Resch KL. Does pentoxifylline prolong the walking distance in exercised claudicants? A placebo-controlled double-blind trial. Angiology 1992;43:121–5.

18. Di Perri T, Guerrini M. Placebo controlled double blind study with pentoxifylline of walking performance in patients with intermittent claudication. Angiology 1983;34:40–5.

19. Green RM, McNamara J. The effects of pentoxifylline on patients with intermittent claudication. J Vasc Surg 1988;7:356–62.

20. Hood SC, Moher D, Barber GG. Management of intermittent claudication with pentoxifylline: meta-analysis of randomized controlled trials. Can Med Assoc J 1996;155:1053–9.

21. Gillings D, Koch G, Reich T, Stager WJ. Another look at the pentoxifylline efficacy data for intermittent claudication. J Clin Pharmacol 1987;27:601–9.

22. Kohda N, Tani T, Nakayama S, et al. Effect of cilostazol, a phosphodiesterase III inhibitor, on experimental thrombosis in the porcine carotid artery. Thromb Res 1999;96:261–8.

23. Igawa T, Tani T, Chijiwa T, et al. Potentiation of anti-platelet aggregating activity of cilostazol with vascular endothelial cells. Thromb Res 1990;57:617–23.

24. Okuda Y, Yukio K, Kamejiro Y. Cilostazol. Cardiovasc Drug Rev 1993;11:451–65.

25. Elam MB, Heckman J, Crouse JR, et al. Effect of the novel antiplatelet agent cilostazol on plasma lipoproteins in patients with intermittent claudication. Arterioscler Thromb Vasc Biol 1998;18:1942–7.

26. Hiatt WR. Medical treatment of peripheral arterial disease and claudication. N Engl J Med 2001;344(21):1608–21.

27. Pletal (cilostazol) product information. Rockville, MD: Otsuka America Pharmaceutical; March 1999.

28. Suri A, Forbes WP, Bramer SL. Pharmacokinetics of multiple-dose oral cilostazol in middle-age and elderly men and women. J Clin Pharmacol 1998;38:141–50.

29. Yoshitomi Y, Kojima S, Sugi T, et al. Antiplatelet treatment with cilostazol after stent implantation. Heart 1999;80:393–6.

30. Packer M, Carver JR, Rodeheffer RJ, et al. Effect of oral milrinone on mortality in severe chronic heart failure. The PROMISE Study Research Group. N Engl J Med 1991;325(21):1468–75.

31. Uretsky BF, Jessup M, Konstam MA, et al. Multicenter trial of oral enoximone in patients with moderate to moderately severe congestive heart failure. Lack of benefit compared with placebo. Enoximone Multicenter Trial Group. Circulation 1990;82(3):774–80.

32. Dawson DL, Cutler BS, Meissner MH, Strandness DE Jr. Cilostazol has beneficial effects in treatment of intermittent claudication: results from a multicenter, randomized, prospective, double-blind trial. Circulation 1998;98:678–86.

33. Money SR, Herd A, Isaacsohn JL, et al. Effect of cilostazol on walking distances in patients with intermittent claudication caused by peripheral vascular disease. J Vasc Surg 1998;27:267–74.

34. Beebe HG, Dawson DL, Cutler BS, et al. A new pharmacological treatment for intermittent claudication: results of a randomized, multicenter trial. Arch Intern Med 1999;159:2041–50.

35. Dawson DL, Cutler BS, Hiatt WR, et al. A comparison of cilostazol and pentoxifylline for treating intermittent claudication. Am J Med 2000;109:523–30.

19

3. ANTIPLATELET THERAPY

Eron D Crouch and Steven R Steinhubl

Introduction

Platelets aggregate with speed and precision at sites of vascular injury as the result of complex interdependent actions of the platelets, vessel wall, and plasma clotting factors. This system is designed to prevent exsanguination when vascular endothelial injury threatens the integrity of the circulatory system. Atherosclerosis causes chronic vascular subendothelial injury and, ultimately, maladaptive inter-luminal platelet aggregation and occlusive clot formation. Peripheral arterial disease (PAD) has been shown to be an independent indicator of more severe systemic atherosclerosis[1] and is thus a risk factor for vascular events. Not surprisingly, antiplatelet therapy is beneficial to a variety of patients with atherosclerosis.[2] The majority of trials have been in patients with cardiovascular and cerebrovascular disease; however, there is substantial evidence that antiplatelet agents also reduce the risk of cerebrovascular and cardiovascular morbidity and mortality in patients with PAD.[2] Other evidence suggests that antiplatelet therapy may also reduce the risk of peripheral arterial occlusive disease (PAOD)[3] and peripheral reocclusion after revascularization.[4] It is important to keep in mind that antiplatelet therapy is only one of several modalities to be used simultaneously in patients with PAD. At the conclusion of this chapter, the reader should: (1) have an overview of the mechanisms of action and key pharmacological features of the different antiplatelet agents; (2) be familiar with several meta-analyses and key clinical trials that provide the evidence for antiplatelet therapy in PAD; and (3) have an evidence-based strategy for choosing antiplatelet agents in common PAD clinical scenarios.

Aspirin

Aspirin is the oldest and most extensively studied antiplatelet agent. By 1944, it was a commonly used analgesic and antipyretic and had been observed to cause excessive bleeding.[5] Shortly thereafter, Paul Gibson proposed that the latter property of aspirin might make it useful for the prevention of coronary thrombosis.[6] Today, there is an overwhelming body of evidence, from clinical trials representing over 100 000 patients, to support aspirin therapy in the primary and secondary prevention of myocardial infarction (MI), stroke, and vascular death in many moderate and high-risk individuals.[7] Patients with PAD (regardless of severity) fall into the 'high-risk' category, because compared with age-matched controls, they have been shown to have a threefold increased rate of cardiovascular mortality.[7]

Mechanism of action

Aspirin is a permanent inhibitor of cyclooxygenase (COX)-1 and COX-2, the isoenzymes responsible for converting arachidonic acid into prostaglandin $(PG)H_2$.[8] This inhibition ultimately results in decreased production of mediators of inflammation (i.e. prostacyclin, PGE_2, and $PGF_{2\alpha}$), as well as thromboxane $(TX)A_2$, an amplifier of platelet aggregation and vasoconstriction (Fig. 3.1).[9] Aspirin is an approximately 50- to 100-fold more potent inhibitor of platelet-derived COX-1 than endothelial cell and monocyte-derived COX-2.[10] This fact partially explains why much lower dosing is required when aspirin is used as an antiplatelet agent versus an analgesic or anti-inflammatory agent.[11]

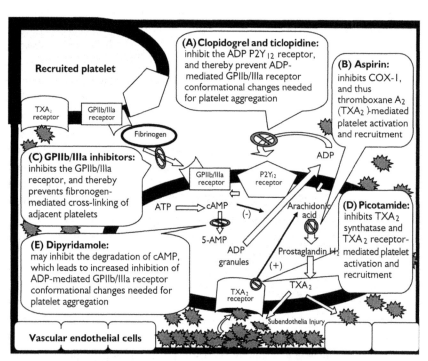

Figure 3.1 *Mechanisms of action of antiplatelet agents. Abbreviations: ADP, adenosine diphosphate; COX-1, cyclooxygenase-1; TXA_2, thromboxane A_2; ATP, adenosine triphosphate; cAMP, cyclic adenosine monophosphate; 5-AMP, 5-adenosine monophosphate, GP, glycoprotein.*

Pharmacokinetics and dosing

Aspirin is rapidly absorbed in the stomach and upper intestines, with peak plasma levels occurring in 30–40 min.[8] Once in the plasma, aspirin is rapidly hydrolyzed to salicylic acid, with plasma levels of the parent compound being essentially undetectable 2–2.5 hours after dosing.[9] Peak plasma levels may take up to 4 hours for enteric-coated tablets.[8] Salicylic acid is primarily metabolized in the liver, in a rate-limiting manner; therefore, the total body clearance decreases at high serum concentrations.[9] A standard dose of aspirin, used as an antiplatelet agent, is 75–325 mg.[9] Enucleated platelets cannot resynthesize COX, as can nucleated monocytes; therefore, once-daily dosing can maintain virtually complete inhibition of platelet TXA_2 production.[8] The platelet inhibitory effect of aspirin last for the life of the platelet, which is approximately 10 days;[8] however, daily dosing is required because approximately 10% of circulating platelets are replaced every 24 hours.[12]

Adverse effects

The ability of aspirin to inhibit PGH_2 accounts for a variety of potential adverse pharmacological effects. The inhibition of PGH_2 leads to decreased production of prostacyclin, PGE_2, and $PGF_{2\alpha}$.[8] Since prostacyclin normally inhibits gastric acid secretion and PGE_2 and $PGF_{2\alpha}$ stimulate production of mucus to protect the endothelium of the stomach and small intestines,[11] inhibition of these mediators can lead to peptic ulcer formation, and gastrointestinal (GI) bleeding. In a meta-analysis of 24 randomized, placebo-controlled trials, representing over 65 000 patients, the incidence of GI hemorrhage was 2.47% for aspirin-treated patients vs 1.42% for those treated with placebo (OR 1.68, 95% CI 1.51–1.88).[13] The risk of GI bleeding appears to be dose-related; however, no commonly used dose is free of risk.[8] Enteric-coated preparations are better tolerated, but have not been shown to decrease the risk of GI bleeding.[14]

Prostacyclin and PGE_2 are also responsible for maintaining glomerular blood flow, by vasodilating the afferent limb of the glomerulus. Inhibition of PGE_2 and prostacyclin by aspirin can lead to afferent limb vasoconstriction and glomerular hypoperfusion, particularly in the presence of efferent limb vasodilators, such as angiotensin-converting enzyme (ACE) inhibitors.[15,16] Fortunately, in the lower doses of aspirin (less than 100 mg) required for platelet inhibition, the risk of this complication is very low.[15]

Clinical trials in peripheral artery disease

In 1985, data from a randomized, double-blind, placebo-controlled trial by Hess and colleagues suggested that aspirin alone or in combination with dipyridamole may delay the need for arterial reconstruction in patients with PAD.[3] Today, the data supporting aspirin therapy to alter the natural course of PAD and decrease the risk of peripheral vascular events is still unclear; however, it is well established that patients with PAD are at an increased risk of MI, stroke, and vascular death and that many of these events can be prevented with aspirin therapy.

The most recent and comprehensive systematic review of the aspirin literature comes from the Antithrombotic Trialists' Collaboration (ATTC) in 2002, which evaluated over 212 000 high-risk patients (representing 287 trials). The ATTC analyzed several doses of aspirin vs placebo in 65 different trials (representing 29 652 vascular events). Overall, aspirin was found to significantly reduce the risk of vascular events by 23%.[2] On direct comparison of different doses of aspirin, no significant difference in vascular events were observed between doses ranging from <75 mg to 1500 mg (Fig. 3.2); however, the risk of GI bleeding did appear to increase in a dose-dependent fashion.[2] ATTC also evaluated over 9700 patients with PAD (representing 42 trials).[2] This meta-analysis showed that antiplatelet therapy provided a 23% odds reduction in serious vascular events ($p = 0.004$); however, once patients were separated by recent history of intermittent claudication, peripheral artery grafting, or peripheral artery angioplasty, the reductions did not reach statistical significance (Fig. 3.3).[2]

Similar benefits had previously been seen in the Antiplatelet Trialists' Collaboration (APTC), which evaluated the use of antiplatelet therapy in over 29 000 high-risk patients (representing 25 trials), including over 21 000 patients treated with some form of aspirin (representing 17 trials). Overall, antiplatelet therapy reduced vascular mortality by 15% and non-fatal stroke or MI by 30%.[17] Although the ATTC analysis included the trials evaluated in APTC, the APTC provided several subgroup analyses of aspirin-treated patients not included in the ATTC. A subset analysis from APTC of approximately 3226 PAD patients with peripheral bypass grafting (saphenous vein or prosthetic) or peripheral artery angioplasty (representing 14 trials)[18] found a 43% odd reduction in vascular occlusion, from 25% in the placebo-treated patients to 16% in the aspirin-treated patients ($p < 0.00001$).[19] A second subset of the APTC, analyzing 3295 patients with intermittent claudication treated with aspirin, found an 18% odds reduction in the risk of MI, stroke, or vascular death (from 11.8% in the control group to 9.7% in the treated group); however, this reduction did not reach clinical significance due to the wide confidence intervals of the risk reduction.[19]

Therapeutic strategies

There is evidence from ATTC and APTC to suggest that PAD patients are at an increased risk of cardiovascular and cerebrovascular events and that many of these events can be prevented by aspirin therapy.[2] In addition, some studies suggest that aspirin may reduce the overall risk of vascular events in patients

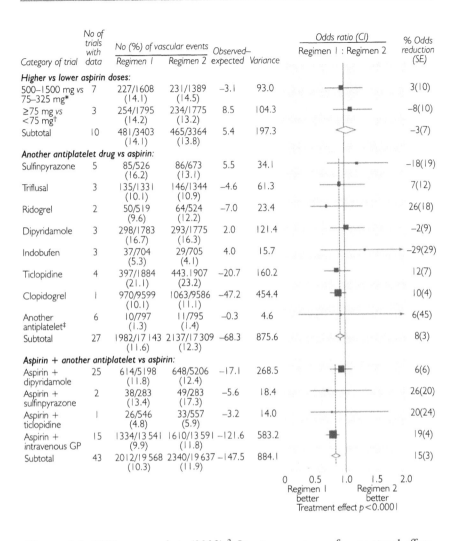

Figure 3.2 *ATTC meta-analysis (2002).*[2] *Direct comparisons of proportional effects of different antiplatelet regimens on vascular events in high-risk patients.*
*Includes one trial comparing 1400 mg/day vs 350 mg/day and another (excluding those with acute stroke) comparing 1000 mg/day vs 300 mg/day among patients who were also given dipyridamole. †Includes two trials comparing 75–325 mg aspirin daily vs <75 mg aspirin daily and one trial of 500–1500 mg aspirin daily vs <75 mg aspirin daily. ‡Includes cilostazol, sulotroban, trapidil, E5510, eptifibatide, and GR32191B. Stratified ratio of odds of an event in regimen 1 group to that in regimen 2 group is plotted for each group of trials (black square) along with its 99% confidence interval (horizontal line). Meta-analysis of results for all trials for a particular comparison (and 95% confidence interval) is represented by an open diamond. (Reproduced with permission of the British Medical Journal 2002; 324:80.)

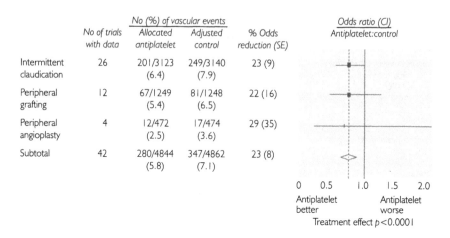

| | No of trials with data | No (%) of vascular events | | % Odds reduction (SE) | Odds ratio (CI) Antiplatelet:control |
		Allocated antiplatelet	Adjusted control		
Intermittent claudication	26	201/3123 (6.4)	249/3140 (7.9)	23 (9)	
Peripheral grafting	12	67/1249 (5.4)	81/1248 (6.5)	22 (16)	
Peripheral angioplasty	4	12/472 (2.5)	17/474 (3.6)	29 (35)	
Subtotal	42	280/4844 (5.8)	347/4862 (7.1)	23 (8)	

0   0.5   1.0   1.5   2.0
Antiplatelet better   Antiplatelet worse
Treatment effect p<0.0001

Figure 3.3: *ATTC meta-analysis (2002).[2] Proportional effects of antiplatelet therapy on vascular events in high-risk patients subdivided by disease category. Stratified ratio of odds of an event in treatment groups to that in control groups is plotted for each group of trials (black square) along with its 99% confidence interval (horizontal line). Meta-analysis of results for all trials (and 95% confidence interval) is represented by an open diamond. Adjusted control totals have been calculated after converting any unevenly randomized trials to even ones by counting control groups more than once, but other statistical calculations are based on actual numbers from individual trials. (Modified from the British Medical Journal 2002;324:78.)*

with intermittent claudication and the risk of (re)occlusion following peripheral artery bypass grafting (Table 3.1).[19] These facts and the low cost of aspirin therapy make it the mainstay of antiplatelet therapy for most patients with PAD. The American College of Chest Physicians (ACCP) Consensus

Table 3.1 Evidence-based antiplatelet therapy in patients with peripheral arterial disease by disease subgroups

Drug	Recommended dose and duration	Evidence
Cardiovascular and cerebrovascular event prevention		
Aspirin	81–325 mg daily for life	APTC: 18% non-significant odds reduction in risk of MI, stroke, or vascular death with aspirin compared to placebo

Table 3.1 (continued)

Drug	Recommended dose and duration	Evidence
Dipyridamole (with aspirin)	Dipyridamole 200 mg AND aspirin 25 mg twice daily for life	ESPS-2: significantly reduced risk of recurrent stroke with dipyridamole and aspirin compared to placebo or aspirin alone; no benefit in CHD ATTC: significant reduction in new vascular events, but to no significant degree more than aspirin alone
Ticlopidine	250 mg twice daily for life	STMS: 30% reduction in mortality with ticlopidine compared to placebo EMATAP: significant reduction in vascular events with ticlopidine compared to placebo
Clopidogrel	75 mg daily for life	CAPRIE: 24% relative risk reduction in MI, stroke, and vascular death with clopidogrel compared to aspirin

Graft patency

Aspirin	81–325 mg daily for life	APTC: 43% proportional reduction in vascular occlusion following peripheral bypass grafting or peripheral artery angioplasty with aspirin compared to placebo
Dipyridamole (with aspirin)	Dipyridamole 200 mg AND aspirin 25 mg twice daily for life	Girolami et al: significant advantage in graft, angioplasty, or endarterectomy patency with dipyridamole and aspirin compared to placebo or vitamin-K inhibitors (i.e. warfarin)
Ticlopidine	250 mg twice daily for up to 2 years	Girolami et al: significantly better patency with ticlopidine compared to placebo for thromboendartectomy or autologous bypass grafting

Table 3.1 (continued)

Drug	Recommended dose and duration	Evidence
Claudication		
Aspirin	325 mg daily for life	Hess et al: possibly delayed need for arterial reconstruction with aspirin compared to placebo
Cilostazol	50–100 mg twice daily for years	ACCP Consensus: 31–47% improvement in walking distances with cilostazol

APTC = Antiplatelet Trialists' Collaboration;[17] ESPS-2 = European Stroke Prevention Study 2;[27,28] ATTC = Antithrombic Trialists' Collaboration;[2] STMS = Swedish Ticlopidine Multicentre Study;[41] EMATAP = Estudio Multicentrico Argentino de la Ticlopidine en las Arteriopatias Perifericas;[42] CAPRIE = Clopidogrel versus Aspirin in Patients at Risk of Ischemic Events;[38] Girolami et al;[4] Hess et al;[3] ACCP = American College of Chest Physicians Consensus.[20]

Group provides the following guidelines for common clinical scenarios in PAD (Table 3.2):[20]

- Aspirin alone (or in combination with dipyridamole) may modify the natural history of intermittent claudication from arteriosclerosis.
- Because patients with intermittent claudication are at high risk of future cardiovascular events (stroke and MI), treat them with lifelong aspirin therapy 81–325 mg/day (or clopidogrel) in the absence of contraindications.
- Use aspirin (81–325 mg/day) in patients having prosthetic, femoropopliteal bypass operations, and antiplatelet therapy should be begun preoperatively.
- Use of lifelong aspirin therapy, 81–325 mg/day, to reduce the incidence of MI and stroke in patients undergoing saphenous vein femoropopliteal or distal bypass.

The recommendations of the ACCP[20] regarding aspirin therapy in patients with PAD are comparable to those of the TransAtlantic Inter-Society Consensus (TASC) Group (Table 3.2).[21–24] Recently, the PAD Antiplatelet Consensus Group created a consensus statement, upgrading the role of clopidogrel and excluding dipyridamole, as a recommended treatment for patients with PAD (Table 3.2). These differences will be discussed later.[25]

Table 3.2 Recommendations for common scenarios in patients with PAD

Scenario	PAD Antiplatelet Consensus Group (2003)	6th ACCP Consensus Group (2001)	TransAtlantic Inter-Society Consensus Group (2000)
Intermittent claudication	• Long-term antiplatelet therapy with ASA 75–325 mg/d OR clopidogrel 75 mg/d.	• ASA alone or in combination with dipyridamole; lifelong ASA therapy (81–325 mg/d) in the absence of contraindications • Clopidogrel may be superior to aspirin and should be considered	• Recommendation 28: All patients with PAD (whether symptomatic or asymptomatic) should be considered for treatment with low-dose aspirin, or other approved antiplatelet (unless contraindicated), to reduce the risk of cardiovascular morbidity and mortality.
Critical/acute limb ischemia		• Systemic anticoagulation with heparin in acute arterial thrombi or emboli; heparin followed by oral anticoagulation to prevent recurrent embolism in patients undergoing thromboembolectomy	
Recurrent vascular events	• Add clopidogrel to ASA OR change ASA to clopidogrel OR change to oral anticoagulant.	N/A	N/A
Patients taking non-aspirin NSAIDs	• DC NSAIDs OR ASA with a PPI OR change ASA to clopidogrel	N/A	
Angioplasty/stenting in peripheral arteries	• Long-term antiplatelet therapy with ASA 75–325 mg/d OR clopidogrel 75 mg/d; stop clopidogrel 5 days before elective surgery		• Recommendation 96: Antiplatelet therapy should be started preoperatively and continued as adjuvant pharmacotherapy after an endovascular or surgical
Peripheral arterial surgical revascularization		• ASA (81–325 mg/d) in patients having prosthetic, femoropopliteal bypass operations, and antiplatelet	

29

Table 3.2 (continued)

Scenario	PAD Antiplatelet Consensus Group (2003)	6th ACCP Consensus Group (2001)	TransAtlantic Inter-Society Consensus Group (2000)
		therapy should be begun preoperatively; addition of dipyridamole (75 mg three times daily) to ASA may provide additional benefit • Lifelong ASA therapy, 81–325 mg/d, in patients undergoing saphenous vein femoropopliteal or distal bypass; clopidogrel in patients unable to take aspirin • Warfarin with or without aspirin after infra-inguinal bypass and other vascular reconstructions; for high-risk patients, combination warfarin and ASA • Do not use antithrombotic therapy for vascular reconstructions involving high-flow, low-resistance arteries >6 mm in diameter in the absence of other indications for antithrombotic therapy; if aspirin indicated for arteriosclerotic disease, then lifelong aspirin therapy in these patients to reduce long-term cardiovascular morbidity and mortality	procedure. Unless subsequently contraindicated, this should be continued indefinitely. Caution should be used in patients in whom use of anticoagulants is proposed.
Abdominal aortic aneurysm	• Antiplatelet therapy		N/A

ASA = acetylsalicylic acid (aspirin); PAD = peripheral arterial disease; NSAIDs = non-steroidal anti-inflammatory drugs; PPI = proton pump inhibitor; N/A = not available, mg/d = mg/day.

Dipyridamole

Dipyridamole was introduced as a treatment for angina in 1961; however, early clinical trials of coronary heart disease (CHD) and stroke demonstrated no clinical benefit from dipyridamole and aspirin over aspirin alone.[26] More recently, the European Stroke Prevention Study 2 (ESPS-2) showed that a long-acting formulation of dipyridamole significantly decreased the risk of recurrent stroke compared with placebo, and that even greater benefit could be gained by a combination of this dipyridamole formulation and aspirin.[27,28] The benefit was not seen in patients with CHD.[27,28] This study led to the Food and Drug Administration (FDA) approval of a combination of 25 mg of aspirin and 200 mg of extended-release dipyridamole (Aggrenox) for use in patients with cerebrovascular ischemic events, but not CHD.[8,29] Due to these mixed results, and the diffuse nature of atherosclerotic disease, the role of dipyridamole (with or without aspirin) for the treatment of PAD remains controversial.

Mechanism of action

The antiplatelet properties of dipyridamole remain unclear; however, it is generally accepted that the agent does prevent platelet phosphodiesterase-mediated degradation of cyclic adenosine monophosphate (c-AMP).[8] This results in increased levels of intracellular c-AMP. Intracellular c-AMP has been shown to inhibit the release of adenosine diphosphate (ADP), which is a known promoter of platelet aggregation (see Fig. 3.1).[11,16] Dipyridamole is also a nonselective vasodilator, which may partially account for the efficacy of this agent, in combination with aspirin, in patients with cerebrovascular disease.[16]

Pharmacokinetics and dosing

Due to the extended absorption phase of dipyridamole, peak plasma levels are achieved 2 hours (range 1–6 hours) after administration of 200 mg twice daily.[29] Dipyridamole is the primary active metabolite, but is conjugated with glucuronic acid in the liver to form monoglucuronide, which has low pharmacodynamic activity. In the steady state, about 80% of the total amount is present as parent compound and 20% as monoglucuronide.[29] While the parent compound remains in circulation, about 95% of the glucuronide metabolite is excreted via bile into the feces, with some evidence of enterohepatic circulation.[8] The alpha half-life (the initial decline following peak concentration) is approximately 40 min, and the beta half-life (the terminal decline in plasma concentration) is approximately 10 hours. Combining dipyridamole with aspirin does not significantly affect the pharmacokinetics of either agent.[29]

Adverse effects

The most common adverse effect leading to discontinuation of dipyridamole is headache, which occurred in approximately 10% of Aggrenox-treated and dipyridamole alone-treated patients in the ESPS-2 trial compared with 3% of those treated with aspirin alone and 4% with placebo.[27,28] Approximately 5% of patients treated with Aggrenox experienced dizziness, and 4% had abdominal pain leading to discontinuation.[29] The incidence of gastrointestinal hemorrhage was 1.2% with Aggrenox, 0.3% with dipyridamole alone, and 0.9% with aspirin alone.[29]

Clinical trials in peripheral artery disease

There are no randomized trials that have specifically evaluated dipyridamole alone for the treatment of PAD; however, its use in combination with aspirin has been studied extensively. In 1994, the APTC analyzed data from 2161 patients with known PAD, using dipyridamole plus aspirin (represented 20 trials) and showed a 40% absolute risk reduction in peripheral arterial (re)occlusion. However, after analyzing only those trials which directly compared the combination of dipyridamole plus aspirin to aspirin alone (951 patients, representing nine trials) there was no significant difference.[18]

In the year 2000, Girolami and colleagues further analyzed this combination in patients with PAD by pooling the results of 10 studies using dipyridamole and aspirin status post peripheral bypass grafting, percutaneous peripheral artery angioplasty, or peripheral endarterectomy (Fig. 3.4).[4] This meta-analysis demonstrated a significant advantage in maintaining patency after peripheral bypass grafting (OR 0.76, 95% CI 0.50–0.85, $p = 0.002$) and after either peripheral artery angioplasty or endarterectomy (OR 0.63, 95% CI 0.40–0.98, $p = 0.04$) with the combination of dipyridamole plus aspirin when compared to placebo or vitamin K inhibitors (i.e. warfarin) (Fig. 3.4).[4] There was no significant decrease in the rate of amputation or mortality (see Fig. 3.4).[4] Unfortunately, this meta-analysis did not directly compare dipyridamole plus aspirin to aspirin alone.

In the 10 404 patients analyzed in ATTC, the combination of dipyridamole and aspirin (represented 25 trials) was also shown to significantly reduce new vascular events (614/5198, 11.8%), but to no significant degree more than aspirin alone (648/5206, 12.4%) (see Fig. 3.2).[2] The reduction in new vascular events was due primarily to a reduced risk of stroke, which was derived mostly from the ESPS-2 trial (6602 patients).[2,27,28]

Therapeutic strategies

Collectively, the literature suggests that the combination of dipyridamole and aspirin does reduce the risk of PAOD in patients with PAD over placebo. In addition, the combination increases the patency rate following peripheral

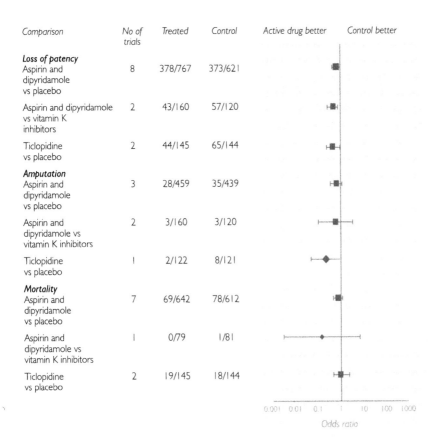

Comparison	No of trials	Treated	Control	Active drug better Control better
Loss of patency				
Aspirin and dipyridamole vs placebo	8	378/767	373/621	
Aspirin and dipyridamole vs vitamin K inhibitors	2	43/160	57/120	
Ticlopidine vs placebo	2	44/145	65/144	
Amputation				
Aspirin and dipyridamole vs placebo	3	28/459	35/439	
Aspirin and dipyridamole vs vitamin K inhibitors	2	3/160	3/120	
Ticlopidine vs placebo	1	2/122	8/121	
Mortality				
Aspirin and dipyridamole vs placebo	7	69/642	78/612	
Aspirin and dipyridamole vs vitamin K inhibitors	1	0/79	1/81	
Ticlopidine vs placebo	2	19/145	18/144	

Odds ratio

Figure 3.4 Girolami et al[4] meta-analysis (2000). Effect of aspirin plus dipyridamole or ticlopidine compared with placebo or vitamin K inhibitors on patency, amputation, and mortality in patients with PAD. Effect of aspirin plus dipyridamole or ticlopidine compared with vitamin K inhibitors or placebo on (loss of) patency, amputation, and mortality in patients with peripheral arterial disease and treated with revascularization procedures. End-of-treatment results are expressed as odds ratio with 95% confidence interval (CI), for individual and combined studies. (Modified from the European Journal of Vascular and Endovascular Surgery 2000;19:374, 377.)

revascularization over placebo or warfarin; however, there are no direct comparisons confirming that the combination of dipyridamole plus aspirin provides added benefit over aspirin alone (see Table 3.1). Consequently, the ACCP Consensus Group provides the following guidelines:

• Aspirin alone or in combination with dipyridamole may modify the natural history of intermittent claudication from arteriosclerosis.[20]

- The addition of dipyridamole to aspirin may provide additional benefit in patients having prosthetic, femoropopliteal bypass operations. Antiplatelet therapy should be begun preoperatively.[20]

Neither the TASC Group nor the PAD Antiplatelet Consensus Group recommends dipyridamole (with or without aspirin) in the treatment of patients with PAD (see Table 3.2).[21–24,25]

Thienopyridines

Ticlopidine, the prototypical thienopyridine, was first introduced as an antiplatelet agent in the 1980s.[30] Today, both ticlopidine and its structural analog clopidogrel have been studied in controlled trials and are thought to be beneficial in the secondary prevention of stroke, MI, and PAOD. Because of its better side-effect profile, clopidogrel is standard of care for the prevention of recurrent ischemic events after coronary percutaneous intervention. It is also often used as an alternative to aspirin in patients with cerebrovascular events. The role of thienopyridines in the treatment of PAD is still evolving.

Mechanism of action

Ticlopidine and clopidogrel are structurally related thienopyridines that inhibit adenosine diphosphate (ADP) binding of the $P2Y_{12}$ receptor, thus inhibiting guanosine 5c-triphosphate-binding protein-mediated downregulation of adenylyl cyclase (see Fig. 3.1).[31–33] The resulting upregulation of adenylyl cyclase prevents conformational changes of the glycoprotein IIb/IIIa receptor needed for high-affinity platelet aggregation (see Fig. 3.1).[11] Thienopyridines do not interact with the arachidonic acid pathways; however, they may have anti-inflammatory properties as evidenced by their ability to lower fibrinogen and C-reactive protein levels.[34,35]

Pharmacokinetics and dosing

Ticlopidine and clopidogrel are rapidly absorbed following oral administration, but subsequently require transformation to an active metabolite by the liver.[36,37] Hepatic metabolism of thienopyridines creates an inherent delay in the maximal antiplatelet effect of approximately 5 hours with a 375 mg loading dose of clopidogrel and up to 7 days with a 500 mg loading dose of ticlopidine. No dose adjustment is necessary for renal-insufficient or elderly patients.[36,37] Approximately 50% of clopidogrel and 60% of ticlopidine is excreted in the urine, with the majority of the remainder being excreted in the feces within 5 days.[36,37] The active metabolite of clopidogrel and ticlopidine forms a covalent, disulfide bond to the platelet $P2Y_{12}$ receptor, and inhibits the receptor for the life of the platelet.[31]

Adverse effects

The most common adverse effects of ticlopidine and clopidogrel are rash and gastrointestinal intolerance.[36,37] In early clinical trials of ticlopidine, these complaints led to discontinuation of the drug in ~20% of patients.[37] Clinical safety data from one large, randomized trial found rash and diarrhea in 6% and 4.5% of patients on clopidogrel, respectively.[38] Much less frequently occurring, but even more concerning, are the blood dyscrasias associated with thienopyridines. Neutropenia has been reported in up to 2.4% of patients receiving ticlopidine,[37] but in only 0.1% of those receiving clopidogrel.[36,37] The latter is comparable to the 0.17% incidence of neutropenia seen in patients receiving aspirin alone.[36,37] Thrombotic thrombocytopenic purpura (TTP) is a particularly worrisome adverse effect of thienopyridines that carries a mortality risk of over 20%. It is estimated to occur in 1 per 1600–4800 patients treated with ticlopidine, but in significantly fewer patients treated with clopidogrel.[39,40] TTP was not seen in clinical trials of over 17 500 clopidogrel-treated patients.[36] In worldwide postmarketing experience, however, TTP has been reported at a rate of about four cases per million clopidogrel-exposed patients.[36] In general, the favorable safety profile of clopidogrel has made it the thienopyridine of choice.

Clinical trials in peripheral artery disease

In 1990, the Swedish Ticlopidine Multicentre Study (STMS) randomized 687 patients with intermittent claudication to ticlopidine or placebo and found that ticlopidine reduced the mortality rate of this high-risk group by 29.1%.[41] Likewise the Estudio Multicentrico Argentino de la Ticlopidine en las Arteriopatias Perifericas (EMATAP) trial (1994) found a significant reduction in vascular events, compared with placebo, by using ticlopidine in 615 patients with intermittent claudication (OR 2.93, 95% CI 0.96–8.99, $p = 0.043$).[42] Neither of these trials specifically evaluated the effects of ticlopidine on peripheral arterial occlusion or revascularization rates. In 2000, Girolami and colleagues analyzed 145 patients (represented two studies) with PAD who underwent thromboendarectomy or autologous saphenous bypass grafting. Patients treated with ticlopidine were found to have significantly better patency when compared to placebo (OR 0.53, 95% CI 0.33–0.85, $p = 0.009$), with a strong trend towards decreased amputation as well (OR 0.29, 95% CI 0.08–1.01, $p = 0.052$) (see Fig. 3.4).[4] There was no significant difference in mortality.[4] In addition, there was no direct comparison of ticlopidine and aspirin in patients with PAD.

In 1996, the Clopidogrel versus Aspirin in Patients at Risk of Ischaemic Events (CAPRIE) trial became the first trial to evaluate clopidogrel vs aspirin in patients with MI, stroke, or PAD. In this study, 19 185 patients were prospectively randomized to clopidogrel or aspirin and found to have a 8.7% relative risk reduction for MI, ischemic stroke, and vascular death with clopidogrel (Table 3.3).[38] Analysis of the CAPRIE-PVD subgroup showed that

Table 3.3 CAPRIE Trial (1996).[38] Treatment effects of clopidogrel vs aspirin on ischemic stroke, myocardial infarction, or vascular death by subgroup

Treatment subgrouped by initial presentation	Recurrent vascular events						
	Stroke	Myocardial infarction	Non-stroke or myocardial infarction vascular death	Total	Event rate per year	Relative risk reduction (95% CI)	p-value
Stroke							
Clopidogrel (nyrs = 6054)	315	44	74	433	7.15%	7.3% (−5.7 to 18.7)	0.26
Aspirin (nyrs = 5979)	338	51	72	461	7.71%		
Myocardial infarction							
Clopidogrel (nyrs = 5787)	42	163	86	291	5.03%	−3.7% (−22.1 to 12.0)	0.66
Aspirin (nyrs = 5843)	42	174	67	283	4.84%		
Peripheral arterial disease							
Clopidogrel (nyrs = 5795)	81	68	66	215	3.71%	23.8% (8.9 to 36.2)	0.0028
Aspirin (nyrs = 5797)	82	108	87	277	4.86%		
All patients							
Clopidogrel (nyrs = 17 636)	438	275	226	939	5.32%	8.7% (0.3 to 16.5)	0.043
Aspirin (nyrs = 17 519)	462	333	226	1021	5.83%		

Source: modified from Lancet 1996;348:1334.

the nearly 6500 patients with known PAD responded even better to clopidogrel (3.71% event rate/year) vs aspirin (4.84% event rate/year) (23.8% relative risk reduction, $p = 0.0028$) (see Table 3.3).[38] The CAPRIE trial did not specifically evaluate clopidogrel's effect on peripheral vascular (re)occlusion or revascularization rates.

There are several ongoing trials that will aid in defining the role of clopidogrel in the treatment of patients with PAD. The Clopidogrel for High Atherothrombotic Risk and Ischemic Stabilization, Management and Avoidance (CHARISMA) trial is a phase III, multicenter, randomized, double-blind study evaluating the rate of vascular events in over 15 000 patients with several risk factors or known CHD, cerebrovascular disease, or PAD. The Clopidogrel and Acetyl Salicylic Acid in Bypass Surgery for Peripheral Arterial Disease (CASPER) trial is a double-blind, randomized study of clopidogrel plus aspirin vs aspirin alone evaluating graft patency and survival in PAD patients undergoing unilateral below-the-knee bypass graft. The Clopidogrel and Aspirin in the Management of Peripheral Endovascular Revascularization (CAMPER) trial is evaluating the effect of clopidogrel plus aspirin vs aspirin alone, in maintaining the patency of lower limb arteries after angioplasty.

Therapeutic strategies

The results of trials such as STMS, EMATAP, Girolami et al and CAPRIE provide support for the use of thienopyridines in patients with PAD. As mentioned earlier, the favorable safety profile of clopidogrel makes it preferable over ticlopidine (see Table 3.1). The ACCP Consensus Group provides the following guideline:

- Clopidogrel may be superior to aspirin in reducing ischemic complications in patients with peripheral vascular disease and intermittent claudication, and should be considered for treatment.[20]

The TASC Group has made no recommendations concerning clopidogrel; however, the PAD Antiplatelet Consensus Group statement, published in 2003, recommends clopidogrel as an alternative to aspirin in high-risk patients (see Table 3.2). In addition, the PAD Antiplatelet Consensus Group provides the options of switching from aspirin to clopidogrel or adding clopidogrel 75 mg once daily to low-dose aspirin in patients with recurrent vascular events, instead of switching to oral anticoagulation (i.e. warfarin), as recommended by the ACCP Consensus Group (2001) (see Table 3.2). Of note, the PAD Antiplatelet Consensus Group recommends stopping clopidogrel for 5 days prior to elective surgery.

Platelet glycoprotein IIb/IIIa receptor antagonists

The first reported glycoprotein IIb/IIIa receptor antagonist (GPIIb/IIIa inhibitor) was a murine antibody developed by Coller and colleagues in 1983.[43] The modern generation of GPIIb/IIIa inhibitors are derived from a number of different sources, but focus on small immunologic molecules or non-immunologic molecules with structural similarities to fibrinogen. Their efficacy and safety as antiplatelet agents, used in conjunction with heparin and aspirin in the setting of acute coronary syndrome (ACS) and coronary angioplasty and stenting, has been supported by several large clinical trials.[2] There are currently three intravenous GPIIb/IIIa inhibitors that are approved by the FDA for this purpose:

1. abciximab (ReoPro),[44] a Fab fragment of a chimeric human–murine antibody
2. tirofiban (Aggrastat),[45] a tyrosine-derived non-peptide that mimics the geometric, stereotactic, and charge characteristics of the GPIIb/IIIa receptor recognition site[8]
3. eptifibatide (Integrillin),[46] a synthetic, non-immunologic, heptapeptide, derived from the structure of the southeastern pigmy rattlesnake venom, barbourin, which recognizes the binding site of GPIIb/IIIa receptors.[47]

These agents are currently under investigation in patients with PAOD as adjunct to thrombolysis.

Mechanism of action

The GPIIb/IIIa receptor is the final common pathway of platelet aggregation. The GPIIb/IIIa receptors on adjacent platelets are cross-linked to each other by a fibrinogen molecule. GPIIb/IIIa inhibitors competitively or non-competitively block these platelet receptors, which essentially eliminates platelet aggregation via fibrinogen cross-linking (see Fig. 3.1).[11]

Pharmacokinetics and dosing

Abciximab, given as an intravenous bolus, rapidly binds to platelet GPIIb/IIIa receptors, decreasing the free plasma concentration of the drug. As a result, the initial half-life is <10 min; and the second-phase half-life is 30 min. With high-dose abciximab, approximately 80% of platelet GPIIb/IIIa receptors are occupied within the first 2 hours. Abciximab is unique from other GPIIb/IIIa inhibitors in that it non-competitively and nearly irreversibly occupies the receptor site. As a result, abciximab can remain platelet-bound in the circulation for 10 or more days.[44]

Tirofiban and eptifibatide both compete with fibrinogen for binding sites on GPIIb/IIIa receptors. As a result, they require high plasma concentrations for adequate inhibition. Both agents also have a short plasma half-life of 2.0–2.5 hours, with platelet function normalizing in <48 hours (see Table 3.1). Both agents are also cleared from the plasma, largely unchanged, by renal excretion. Therefore, renal dose adjustment is mandatory in renal-insufficient patients.[45,46]

Adverse effects

The risk of major hemorrhage from the combination of intravenous GPIIb/IIIa inhibitors, heparin, and aspirin is only slightly more than that seen with a combination of heparin and aspirin alone (4.0% vs 3.0%, respectively, $p =$ NS); nevertheless, this is significantly greater than placebo.[48] The incidence of intracranial hemorrhage is approximately 0.3%. Transient thrombocytopenia (platelet count <100 000/mm^3) is another important adverse effect of GPIIb/IIIa inhibitors, in particular abciximab, occurring in approximately 2–3% of patients.[49] It is associated with an increased risk of bleeding,[50] and occasionally with a paradoxically increased risk of thrombosis.[51] The platelet count should be monitored prior to treatment, 2–4 hours following the initial bolus, then daily.[44,45]

Clinical trials in peripheral artery disease

As mentioned above, the majority of evidence for the safety and efficacy of GPIIb/IIIa inhibitors comes from the cardiovascular literature. The ATTC evaluated over 24 000 high-risk patients with acute coronary syndromes (represented 15 trials) randomized to a GPIIb/IIIa inhibitor plus aspirin vs aspirin alone and found that the combination of a GPIIb/IIIa inhibitor plus aspirin proportionally reduced vascular events by 19% compared to aspirin alone ($p = 0.0001$) (see Fig. 3.2).[2] This proportional reduction was larger among patients with acute coronary syndrome (ACS) undergoing percutaneous intervention (PCI) (32% with GPIIb/IIIa inhibitor plus aspirin vs 12% with aspirin alone; $p = 0.003$), but still statistically significant among those that did not undergo PCI ($p = 0.02$).[2] There were few intracranial hemorrhages in both groups (0.2% vs 0.1%).[2]

There have been no large, randomized trials evaluating GPIIb/IIIa inhibitors in patients with PAD; however, recently, several small trials, representing over 300 patients, have shown promising results using GPIIb/IIIa inhibitors as adjunct to catheter-directed thrombolytic therapy for PAOD (see Table 3.2).[52–58] Schweizer and colleagues (2000) conducted a pilot study to evaluate the use of abciximab vs aspirin in conjunction with thrombolysis in 84 patients with acute peripheral arterial thrombosis. All patients were given intravenous t-PA (tissue plasminogen activator) and 500 IU heparin/hour, and then randomized to either aspirin or a bolus of abciximab 0.25 mg/kg followed by 10 µg/min over 12 hours (heparin reduced to 250 IU/h).[52] Compared to aspirin, adjunctive use of abciximab reduced the rates of rehospitalization

(14% vs 10%, respectively), reinterventions (11% vs 9% respectively), and amputations (5% vs 3%, respectively) (summed, inter-group difference $p <0.05$).[52] There were no major bleeding complications.[52] In 2003, Schweizer and colleagues also published a study of 60 patients with PAOD receiving catheter-directed thrombolysis plus abciximab or tirofiban and found similar efficacy and safety between the two GPIIb/IIIa inhibitors.[56] Eptifibatide has also shown promising results used in conjunction with catheter-directed TNK (tenecteplase) for PAOD.[57] In early 2004, preliminary results from the prospective RELAX trial were published, evaluating the safety and efficacy of four different doses of catheter-based intra-arterial t-PA monotherapy vs intra-arterial t-PA plus intravenous abciximab combination therapy in patients with acute or subacute peripheral arterial occlusive disease.[58] Overall, t-PA doses of at least 0.2 U/h were effective at dissolving thrombus and restoring patency.[58] There was no clear dose–response relationship. When compared to t-PA monotherapy, the addition of intravenous abciximab to t-PA was associated with a decreased occurrence of distal embolic events requiring intervention (31% vs 5%, respectively; $p = 0.014$), without a significant increase in the risk of hemorrhagic complications (15% vs 20%, respectively).[58] There were no intracranial hemorrhagic events in the 74 t-PA-treated patients (38 patients received abciximab).[58] Over the range of t-PA doses studied for peripheral arterial thrombolysis, there were no significant differences in safety or efficacy.[58]

Therapeutic strategies
Although preliminary results of several recent trials have been promising, further investigation is still needed to define the role of GPIIb/IIIa inhibitors in catheter-directed thrombolysis for PAOD. Current guidelines make no recommendations concerning the use of GPIIb/IIIa inhibitors in PAD.

Other antiplatelet agents

Cilostazol (Pletal) is a peripheral vasodilator and phosphodiesterase inhibitor with antiplatelet properties similar to dipyridamole.[59] The results of eight randomized, placebo-controlled, double-blind trials suggest that patients treated with cilostazol, 50–100 mg given twice daily, have statistically significant improvements in walking distances when compared to patients treated with placebo.[59] The effect of cilostazol on walking distance has been seen as early as after 2 weeks of treatment.[59] As a result of these findings, cilostazol is FDA-approved for the treatment of intermittent claudication. This agent is discussed in detail in Chapter 2.

Picotamide is a TXA_2 receptor inhibitor which also inhibits thromboxane synthetase-mediated platelet activation. It has shown promise in reducing vascular events in a variety of high-risk patients, when compared to placebo (see Fig. 3.1);[20] however, it has not been directly compared to aspirin or clopidogrel, two proven antiplatelet agents.

Several other experimental antiplatelet agents have been evaluated in patients with CHD, cerebrovascular disease, and PAD, including sulfinpyrazone, suloctidil, sulotroban, trifusal, ridogrel, and indobufen.[2] None of these agents have been proven to reduce vascular events when compared with aspirin (see Fig. 3.2).

Conclusion

Platelets play an essential role in vascular hemostasis; however, in the setting of atherosclerotic PAD, they contribute to pathologic thrombosis. This is associated with significant morbidity and mortality. Antiplatelet therapy is an important part of management of these patients, not only to reduce the risk of PAOD and increase patency rate after revascularization but also, more importantly, to decrease these patient's high risk of cerebrovascular and cardiovascular events.

Key points

- Compared with age-matched controls, patients with PAD have been shown to have a threefold increased rate of cardiovascular mortality.[7]
- Aspirin alone (or in combination with dipyridamole) may modify the natural history of intermittent claudication from arteriosclerosis.[20]
- Because patients with intermittent claudication are at high risk of future cardiovascular events (stroke and MI), treat them with lifelong aspirin therapy, 81–325 mg daily (or clopidogrel), in the absence of contraindications.[20]
- Although the combination of dipyridamole plus aspirin has been shown to decrease the risk of recurrent strokes,[27,28] there are no direct comparisons confirming that the combination provides added benefit over aspirin alone in the treatment of PAD or CHD.
- Clopidogrel (with and without aspirin) has proven benefit over aspirin in the treatment of CHD and stroke and may be superior to aspirin in reducing ischemic complications in patients with PAD and intermittent claudication.[20]
- The role of clopidogrel in the treatment of PAD is still evolving.
- Although preliminary results of several recent trials have been promising,[52–58] further investigation is still needed to define the role of GPIIb/IIIa inhibitors in catheter-directed thrombolysis for PAOD.

References

1. Criqui MH, Denenberg JO, Langer RD, Fronek A. The epidemiology of peripheral arterial disease: importance of identifying the population at risk. Vasc Med 1997;2:221–6.

2. Antithrombotic Trialists' Collaboration. Collaborative meta-analysis of randomised trials of antiplatelet therapy for prevention of death, myocardial infarction, and stroke in high risk patients. BMJ 2002;324:71–86.

3. Hess H, Mietaschk A, Deichsel G. Drug-induced inhibition of platelet function delays progression of peripheral occlusive arterial disease. A prospective double-blind arteriographically controlled trial. Lancet 1985;1:415–19.

4. Girolami B, Bernardi E, Prins MH, et al. Antiplatelet therapy and other interventions after revascularisation procedures in patients with peripheral arterial disease: a meta-analysis. Eur J Vasc Endovasc Surg 2000;19:370–80.

5. Quick AJ. Salicylates and hemorrhage. JAMA 1944;126:1167.

6. Gibson P. Salicylic acid for coronary thrombosis? Lancet 1948;1:965.

7. Robless P, Mikhailidis DP, Stansby G. Systematic review of antiplatelet therapy for the prevention of myocardial infarction, stroke or vascular death in patients with peripheral vascular disease. Br J Surg 2001;88:787–800.

8. Patrono C, Coller B, Dalen JE, et al. Platelet-active drugs: the relationships among dose, effectiveness, and side effects. Chest 2001;119:39S–63S.

9. Aspirin. Physicians' Desk Reference (PDR) Electronic Library, 2004.

10. Cipollone F, Patrignani P, Greco A, et al. Differential suppression of thromboxane biosynthesis by indobufen and aspirin in patients with unstable angina. Circulation 1997;96:1109–16.

11. Schafer AI, Ali NM, Levine GN. Hemostasis, thrombosis, fibrinolysis, and cardiovascular disease. In: Braunwald E, Zipes DP, Libby P, eds. Heart disease: a textbook of cardiovascular medicine, 6th edn. Philadelphia: WB Saunders Co; 2001:2099–132.

12. Cerskus AL, Ali M, Davies BJ, McDonald JW. Possible significance of small numbers of functional platelets in a population of aspirin-treated platelets in vitro and in vivo. Thromb Res 1980;18:389–97.

13. Derry S, Loke YK. Risk of gastrointestinal haemorrhage with long term use of aspirin: meta-analysis. BMJ 2000;321:1183–7.

14. Hoftiezer JW, Silvoso GR, Burks M, Ivey KJ. Comparison of the effects of regular and enteric-coated aspirin on gastroduodenal mucosa of man. Lancet 1980;2:609–12.

15. Becker RC, Fintel DJ, Green D. Antithrombotic therapy, 2nd edn. New York: Professional Communications Inc; 2002:63–76.

16. Mycek MJ, Harvey RA, Champe PC. Lippincott's illustrated reviews: pharmacology, 2nd edn. Philadelphia: Lippincott Williams & Wilkins; 1992:401–11.

17. Secondary prevention of vascular disease by prolonged antiplatelet treatment. Antiplatelet Trialists' Collaboration. Br Med J (Clin Res Ed) 1988;296:320–31.

18. Collaborative overview of randomised trials of antiplatelet therapy – II: Maintenance of vascular graft or arterial patency by antiplatelet therapy. Antiplatelet Trialists' Collaboration. BMJ 1994;308:159–68.

19. Hiatt WR. Preventing atherothrombotic events in peripheral arterial disease: the use of antiplatelet therapy. J Intern Med 2002;251:193–206.

20. Jackson MR, Clagett GP. Antithrombotic therapy in peripheral arterial occlusive disease. Chest 2001;119:283S–299S.

21. Management of peripheral arterial disease (PAD). TransAtlantic Inter-Society Consensus (TASC). Section D: chronic critical limb ischaemia. Eur J Vasc Endovasc Surg 2000;19 (Suppl A):S144–243.

22. Management of peripheral arterial disease (PAD). TransAtlantic Inter-Society Consensus (TASC). Section C: acute limb ischaemia. Eur J Vasc Endovasc Surg 2000;19 (Suppl A):S115–43.

23. Management of peripheral arterial disease (PAD). TransAtlantic Inter-Society Consensus (TASC). Eur J Vasc Endovasc Surg 2000; 19 (Suppl A):Si-xxviii, S1–250.

24. Management of peripheral arterial disease (PAD). TransAtlantic Inter-Society Consensus (TASC). Section B: intermittent claudication. Eur J Vasc Endovasc Surg 2000; 19 (Suppl A):S47–114.

25. Antiplatelet therapy in peripheral arterial disease. Consensus statement. Eur J Vasc Endovasc Surg 2003;26:1–16.

26. FitzGerald GA. Dipyridamole. N Engl J Med 1987;316:1247–57.

27. Diener HC, Cunha L, Forbes C, et al. European Stroke Prevention Study. 2. Dipyridamole and acetylsalicylic acid in the secondary prevention of stroke. J Neurol Sci 1996;143:1–13.

28. Forbes CD. European Stroke Prevention Study: 2. Dipyridamole and acetylsalicylic acid in the secondary prevention of stroke. Int J Clin Pract 1997;51:205–8.

29. Dipyridamole/Aspirin (Aggrenox). Physicians' Desk Reference (PDR) Electronic Library, 2004.

30. Gent M. The Canadian American Ticlopidine Study (CATS) in thromboembolic stroke. Lancet 1989;1:1216–20.

31. Ding Z, Kim S, Dorsam RT, Jin J, Kunapuli SP. Inactivation of the human P2Y12 receptor by thiol reagents requires interaction with both extracellular cysteine residues, Cys17 and Cys270. Blood 2003;101:3908–14.

32. Conley PB, Delaney SM. Scientific and therapeutic insights into the role of the platelet P2Y12 receptor in thrombosis. Curr Opin Hematol 2003;10:333–8.

33. Herbert JM, Savi P. P2Y12, a new platelet ADP receptor, target of clopidogrel. Semin Vasc Med 2003;3:113–22.

34. de Maat MP, Arnold AE, van Buuren S, Wilson JH, Kluft C. Modulation of plasma fibrinogen levels by ticlopidine in healthy volunteers and patients with stable angina pectoris. Thromb Haemost 1996;76:166–70.

35. Vivekananthan DP, Bhatt DL, Chew DP, et al. Effect of clopidogrel pretreatment on periprocedural rise in C-reactive protein after percutaneous coronary intervention. Am J Cardiol 2004;94:358–60.

36. Clopidigrel (Plavix). Physicians' Desk Reference (PDR) Electronic Library, 2004.

37. Ticlopidine (Ticlid). Physicians' Desk Reference (PDR) Electronic Library, 2004.

38. A randomised, blinded, trial of clopidogrel versus aspirin in patients at risk of ischaemic events (CAPRIE). CAPRIE Steering Committee. Lancet 1996;348:1329–39.

39. Bennett CL, Kiss JE, Weinberg PD, et al. Thrombotic thrombocytopenic purpura after stenting and ticlopidine. Lancet 1998;352:1036–7.

40. Steinhubl SR, Tan WA, Foody JM, Topol EJ. Incidence and clinical course of thrombotic thrombocytopenic purpura due to ticlopidine following coronary stenting. EPISTENT Investigators. Evaluation of Platelet IIb/IIIa Inhibitor for Stenting. JAMA 1999;281:806–10.

41. Janzon L. Prevention of myocardial infarction and stroke in patients with intermittent claudication; effects of ticlopidine. Results from STIMS, the Swedish Ticlopidine Multicentre Study. J Intern Med 1990;227:301–8.

42. Blanchard J. Results of EMATAP: a double-blind placebo-controlled multicentre trial of ticlopidine in patients with peripheral arterial disease. Nouv Rev Fr Hematol 1994;35:523–8.

43. Coller BS, Peerschke EI, Scudder LE, Sullivan CA. A murine monoclonal antibody that completely blocks the binding of fibrinogen to platelets produces a thrombasthenic-like state in normal platelets and binds to glycoproteins IIb and/or IIIa. J Clin Invest 1983;72:325–38.

44. Abciximab (ReoPro). Physicians' Desk Reference (PDR) Electronic Library, 2004.

45. Tirofiban (Aggrastat). Physicians' Desk Reference (PDR) Electronic Library, 2004.

46. Eptifibatide (Integrillin). Physicians' Desk Reference (PDR) Electronic Library, 2004.

47. Scarborough RN, Naughton MA, Teng W, et al. Design of potent and specific integrin antagonists. Peptide antagonists with high specificity for the glycoprotein IIb-IIIa. J Biol Chem 1993;268:1066–73.

48. Inhibition of the platelet glycoprotein IIb/IIIa receptor with tirofiban in unstable angina and non-Q-wave myocardial infarction. Platelet Receptor Inhibition in Ischemic Syndrome Management in Patients Limited by Unstable Signs and Symptoms (PRISM-PLUS) Study Investigators. N Engl J Med 1998;338:1488–97.

49. Giugliano RP. Drug-Induced Thrombocytopenia: Is it a serious concern for glycoprotein IIb/IIIa receptor inhibitors? J Thromb Thrombolysis 1998;5:191–202.

50. Berkowitz SD, Sane DC, Sigmon KN, et al. Occurrence and clinical significance of thrombocytopenia in a population undergoing high-risk percutaneous coronary revascularization. Evaluation of c7E3 for the Prevention of Ischemic Complications (EPIC) Study Group. J Am Coll Cardiol 1998;32:311–19.

51. Mahaffey KW, Harrington RA, Simoons ML, et al. Stroke in patients with acute coronary syndromes: incidence and outcomes in the platelet glycoprotein IIb/IIIa in unstable angina. Receptor Suppression Using Integrilin Therapy (PURSUIT) trial. The PURSUIT Investigators. Circulation 1999;99:2371–7.

52. Schweizer J, Kirch W, Koch R, et al. Short- and long-term results of abciximab versus aspirin in conjunction with thrombolysis for patients with peripheral occlusive arterial disease and arterial thrombosis. Angiology 2000;51:913–23.

53. Drescher P, Crain MR, Rilling WS. Initial experience with the combination of reteplase and abciximab for thrombolytic therapy in peripheral arterial occlusive disease: a pilot study. J Vasc Interv Radiol 2002;13:37–43.

54. Rocha-Singh KJ, Trokey J. Combined glycoprotein IIb/IIIa receptor inhibition and low-dose fibrinolysis for peripheral arterial thrombosis. Catheter Cardiovasc Interv 2002;55:457–60.

55. Drescher P, McGuckin J, Rilling WS, Crain MR. Catheter-directed thrombolytic therapy in peripheral artery occlusions: combining reteplase and abciximab. AJR Am J Roentgenol 2003;180:1385–91.

56. Schweizer J, Kirch W, Koch R, et al. Use of abciximab and tirofiban in patients with peripheral arterial occlusive disease and arterial thrombosis. Angiology 2003;54:155–61.

57. Burkart DJ, Borsa JJ, Anthony JP, Thurlo SR. Thrombolysis of acute peripheral arterial and venous occlusions with tenecteplase and eptifibatide: a pilot study. J Vasc Interv Radiol 2003;14:729–33.

58. Ouriel K, Castaneda F, McNamara T, et al. Reteplase monotherapy and reteplase/abciximab combination therapy in peripheral arterial occlusive disease: results from the RELAX trial. J Vasc Interv Radiol 2004;15:229–38.

59. Cilostazol (Pletal). Physicians' Desk Reference (PDR) Electronic Library, 2004.

4. LIPID-MODIFYING THERAPY

Victor M Mejia and Herbert D Aronow

Association between dyslipidemia and atherosclerotic vascular disease

The association between increased serum cholesterol and coronary artery disease (CAD) is well established. The Framingham Study and the Multiple Risk Factor Intervention Trial (MRFIT) found that the incidence of coronary events rose with increasing cholesterol levels.[1–3] Dyslipidemia is also linked to the development and clinical manifestations of peripheral arterial disease (PAD).[4,5] In the Framingham study, the odds ratio for claudication increased by 1.2 with each 40 mg/dL increment in total cholesterol.[6] Similarly, elevated total cholesterol and triglyceride levels and decreased HDL levels were associated with PAD in age- and sex-adjusted analyses from the Framingham Offspring Study;[7] the odds of PAD increased by 10% with each 5 mg/dL decrement in HDL. In the Cardiovascular Health Study (CHS),[8] increasing total and LDL cholesterol and triglycerides and decreasing HDL cholesterol levels were related to decreasing ankle–brachial index (ABI) in a randomly selected sample of Medicare participants. These associations have been corroborated in the Strong Heart Study,[9] the Honolulu Heart Program,[10] and the Edinburgh Artery Study.[11] Interestingly, the relation between increasing non-HDL cholesterol and a lower ABI was even stronger in current smokers than in former or non-smokers in CHS.

Non-pharmacological lipid modification and stable cardiovascular disease

One of the first randomized studies to link improved cardiovascular outcomes with lipid lowering was the Program on the Surgical Control of the Hyperlipidemias (POSCH).[12] This trial enrolled 838 patients with a prior myocardial infarction (MI) and elevated serum cholesterol. Participants were randomized to partial ileal bypass or to no surgery. At 5 years, the surgical group had 23.3% lower total plasma cholesterol and 37.7% lower LDL cholesterol than the control group. While there was no difference in overall survival, surgery significantly reduced the combined end point of death due to

CAD and non-fatal MI (19.5% vs 30%, relative risk reduction (RRR) 65%, p <0.001).[12] Interestingly, PAD or intermittent claudication developed less frequently in the surgical group (12.4% vs 17%, RRR 27%, p = 0.038).[12]

Statins and stable cardiovascular disease

Several large randomized trials have shown that 3-hydroxy-3-methyl-glutaryl-coenzyme A reductase inhibitors (statins) reduce the incidence of non-fatal MI, hospitalization for unstable angina, revascularization procedures, and both cardiovascular and total mortality in patients with CAD.[12–17] More recent trials have confirmed these benefits in patients with PAD (Table 4.1). The Scandinavian Simvastatin Survival Study (4S) examined whether statin therapy in patients with stable CAD and increased cholesterol levels improved survival.[15] This study randomized 4444 patients with a history of MI and total serum cholesterol above 212 mg/dL to simvastatin (titrated to reduce serum total cholesterol to <201 mg/dL) or placebo and followed them over a median of more than 5 years. At baseline, 6% of patients in each group reported claudication. Most patients in the simvastatin group (72%) achieved target cholesterol levels (<201 mg/dL) after 1 year of therapy. Simvastatin significantly reduced LDL cholesterol compared to placebo.[15] Importantly, simvastatin significantly reduced overall mortality, the first lipid-modifying trial to do so, a benefit that was largely driven by a reduction in coronary death that became apparent after 1 year of therapy.

Most patients with CAD have cholesterol levels that are not markedly elevated.[2,18] The Cholesterol and Recurrent Events (CARE) Trial studied the effectiveness of statin therapy in subjects with stable CAD, a history of MI and average cholesterol levels (total plasma cholesterol <240 mg/dL and LDL cholesterol of 115–174 mg/dL).[17] Patients were randomized to pravastatin 40 mg daily or placebo. At baseline, 12.9% of subjects had diffuse atherosclerotic disease, defined as lower extremity (8.5% of cohort) or cerebrovascular atherosclerosis or symptomatic claudication by the Rose questionnaire.[19]

Pravastatin significantly reduced mean LDL by 28% (p <0.001) and the incidence of death from CAD or symptomatic MI when compared with placebo (13.2% vs 10.2%, RRR 24%, p = 0.003).[17] Pravastatin's benefit was dependent upon baseline LDL level, with a greater benefit observed in patients with higher baseline LDL (31% vs 21%, RRR 35%, p = 0.008 in patients with baseline LDL >150 mg/dL; 27% vs 20%, RRR 26%, p <0.001 in patients with baseline LDL 125–150 mg/dL). Pravastatin therapy did not improve overall survival, but significantly reduced the rate of stroke (3.8% vs 2.6%, RRR 31%, p = 0.03), a pre-specified end point.

The Long-Term Intervention with Pravastatin in Ischemic Disease (LIPID) study was initiated in 1989 to better define the effect of statin therapy on outcomes in patients with CAD over a broad range of cholesterol levels.[14] Patients with a history of MI or unstable angina and a total cholesterol level between 155 and 271 mg/dL were eligible. Claudication and history of stroke were present in 10% and 4% of enrolled patients, respectively. Subjects were randomized to pravastatin 40 mg daily or placebo and followed for 6.1 years.

Pravastatin reduced the rate of death from CAD by 24% compared with placebo (8.3% vs 6.4%, RRR 24% [95% CI 12–35%], $p <0.001$).[16] Pravastatin also significantly reduced overall mortality by 22% compared with placebo (14.1% vs 11.0%, RRR 22% [95% CI 13–31%], $p <0.001$). The incidence of MI, death due to CAD, surgical or percutaneous coronary revascularization, and stroke were significantly lower in the pravastatin group, with risk reductions ranging from 19 to 29%.[14] Unlike CARE, a benefit in patients with lower cholesterol levels (LDL levels below 135 mg/dL) was apparent in LIPID; pravastatin reduced the risk of CAD death and non-fatal MI by 16% in this cohort. LIPID also provided evidence of benefit among patients with a history of unstable angina, a group not enrolled in the 4S or CARE trials.

The Heart Protection Study (HPS) focused on treating patients at elevated cardiovascular risk largely independent of cholesterol levels in both primary and secondary prevention settings. Candidates were required to be at an increased 5-year risk of death from coronary heart disease because of a history of CAD, occlusive disease of non-coronary arteries, or diabetes.[13] A total of 20 536 patients were randomized to simvastatin 40 mg daily or placebo. Of the 13 386 with a history of CAD, 1460 had cerebrovascular disease and 4047 had PAD. Among the 7150 patients without coronary disease, 1820 patients had cerebrovascular disease and 2701 had PAD.[13] The primary end point was all-cause mortality and CAD death.

Over 5 years of follow-up, total and LDL cholesterol were 46.4 mg/dL and 38.7 mg/dL lower, respectively, in the simvastatin- than placebo-treated patients.[13] Simvastatin also significantly reduced all-cause mortality (12.9% vs 14.7%, RRR 13% [95% CI 6–19%], $p = 0.0003$). This reduction was mainly due to an 18% reduction in the coronary death rate (6.9% vs 5.7%, $p = 0.0005$).[13] Simvastatin also reduced the composite end point of non-fatal MI or coronary death by 27% (11.8% vs 8.7%, RRR 27% [95% CI 21–33%], $p <0.0001$) and coronary revascularization by 30% (7.1% vs 5.0%, $p <0.0001$) compared with placebo. As in other trials of patients at risk for or with clinically stable CAD, the improved outcomes became evident after approximately 1 year of therapy.

As in LIPID, the benefit of statin therapy was consistent across a broad range of cholesterol levels. HPS was the first major trial to show significant

Table 4.1 Secondary prevention lipid-lowering trials

	4S	CARE	LIPID	HPS
Patient population	Men and women aged 35–70 with history of acute MI or angina	Men and women aged 21–75 with history of acute MI, LDL 115–174 mg/dL and total cholesterol < 240 mg/dL	Men and women aged 31–75 with history of acute MI or USA	Men and women aged 40–80 with high 5-year cardiovascular risk
Study duration, years	5.4	5	6.1	5
Number of patients	4444	4159	9014	20536
Baseline LDL[1]	188 mg/dL	139 mg/dL	150 mg/dL	130 mg/dL
Statin dose	Simvastatin 20–40 mg	Pravastatin 40 mg	Pravastatin 40 mg	Simvastatin 40 mg
Reduction in LDL[2]	35%	32%	25%	38%
Primary end point	Total mortality	Death from CAD or non-fatal MI	Death from CAD	Total mortality, death from CAD or death from non-CAD
Major coronary events[3]	RR = 0.66, [95% CI 0.59–0.75], p <0.00001	RR = 0.76, [95% CI NA[4]], p = 0.003	RR = 0.76, [NA], p <0.001	RR = 0.73, [95% CI 0.67–0.79], p <0.0001
Coronary mortality	RR = 0.58, [95% CI 0.46–0.73], p(NA)	RR = 0.80, [95% CI NA], p = 0.10	RR = 0.76, [NA], p <0.001	RR = 0.82, [95% CI NA], p <0.0001
Total mortality	RR = 0.7, [95% CI 0.58–0.85], p = 0.0003	RR = 0.91, [95% CI NA], p = 0.37	RR = 0.78, [NA], p <0.001	RR = 0.87, [95% CI 0.81–0.94], p = 0.0003

1 Reported as the median value in LIPID and the mean value in the other studies.
2 Reported as percent change from baseline in 4S and CARE, percent change compared to placebo in LIPID, and absolute difference compared to placebo in HPS.
3 Major coronary events were defined as death due to CAD or non-fatal MI.
4 NA = Not available or reported.

risk reductions in patients with LDL levels below 100 mg/dL at baseline. Somewhat surprisingly, among 3500 subjects with a baseline LDL below 100 mg/dL, reducing the mean LDL from 97 mg/dL in the placebo group to 65 mg/dL in the simvastatin group produced a risk reduction in line with that observed in patients with much higher baseline LDL levels.

HPS enrolled patients according to high-risk disease categories and reported outcomes accordingly. For patients with a history of cerebrovascular disease, treatment with simvastatin led to a lower risk of a major vascular events than in placebo-treated patients with (37.4% vs 32.4%, p <0.0001) or without a history of CAD (23.6% vs 18.7%, p <0.0001). The incidence of a first major coronary event was also significantly lower in simvastatin- than in placebo-treated patients with cerebrovascular disease (13.3% vs 10.4%, p <0.0001). Patients with PAD also fared better with simvastatin than placebo. The rate of first major vascular events (32.7% vs 26.4%, p <0.0001) and first major coronary events (13.8% vs 10.9%, p <0.0001) in this cohort was significantly lower in the simvastatin than in the placebo group, respectively.[13] These differences were observed among patients with and without CAD at baseline.

In patients with PAD, simvastatin reduced the incidence of non-coronary revascularization by 16% (5.2% vs 4.4%, RRR 16% [95% CI 5–26%], p = 0.006). Allocation to simvastatin also yielded a 25% relative reduction in the rate of new strokes (5.7% vs 4.3%, RRR 25% [95% CI 15–34%], p <0.0001).

HPS also enrolled 5963 diabetic subjects.[20–22] Among this high-risk group, 1070 (18%) had a history of non-coronary vascular disease. Treatment of diabetic patients with simvastatin produced a significant reduction in peripheral macrovascular complications (6.5% vs 5.2%, p = 0.03). These complications included any peripheral artery surgery (2.2% vs 1.3%, respectively), peripheral angioplasty (2.3% vs 1.9%, respectively), leg amputation (2.2% vs 2.2%, respectively), or leg ulcer (1.5% vs 1.3%, respectively).[23] Prior trials of statin therapy yielded conflicting results regarding the effect of statin therapy on the incidence of stroke, primarily because some of these were underpowered to do so.[13,15,24–26] HPS was designed to assess the effects of aggressive statin therapy on stroke incidence. Treatment with simvastatin was associated with a significant 25% reduction (p <0.0001) in the rate of stroke, which was mainly due to a 30% reduction in the rate of ischemic stroke.[27] There was also a highly significant reduction in the rate of stroke among patients without a history of CAD treated with simvastatin.[27] Unlike the data from the PROspective Study of Pravastatin in the Elderly at Risk (PROSPER) trial, which did not show a reduction in the rate of stroke among high-risk elderly patients after 3 years of treatment with pravastatin,[28] the preventive benefit in the incidence of stroke was seen after 1 year in HPS, similar to the effect on coronary risk reduction.

There are no published randomized placebo-controlled statin trials solely comprising PAD patients that examine cardiovascular outcomes. In an observational study, Schillinger et al examined patients with angiographically proven PAD admitted to the angiology service of a tertiary care university hospital for a percutaneous procedure. At baseline, patients on statin therapy had ABIs similar to those not taking statins (overall median ABI 0.51), but the non-statin group had significantly more critical limb ischemia (27% vs 14%, p <0.001).[29] Multivariate analysis revealed an interaction between statins and the degree of systemic inflammation, with a lower risk of death (adjusted hazard ratio reduction (HRR) 42% [95% CI 1–67%], p = 0.046) or the composite of MI and death (adjusted HRR 54% [95% CI 13–75%], p = 0.016) seen with statin therapy when the hs-CRP (highly sensitive C-reative protein) level was greater than 0.42 mg/dL, but no improvement in survival when the level of hs-CRP was below this threshold. These cardiovascular outcome data are consistent with those from PAD patients enrolled in the 4S, LIPID, CARE, and HPS trials.

Statins in acute coronary syndromes

Despite the established benefit of statins in patients with CAD, most studies excluded patients with unstable angina and did not enroll patients until 3–6 months after a qualifying coronary event.[14,15,17] Early large-scale observational data suggested that statins significantly reduced adverse cardiovascular outcomes when initiated soon after an acute coronary syndrome.[30] The Myocardial Ischemia Reduction with Aggressive Cholesterol Lowering (MIRACL) study was the first randomized trial to examine this question. MIRACL randomized patients with unstable angina or an acute non-Q-wave MI within 24–96 hours to atorvastatin 80 mg or placebo daily for 16 weeks. The primary end point was a combination of death, non-fatal acute MI, cardiac arrest, or recurrent symptomatic myocardial ischemia. A total of 3086 patients were enrolled, and included 266 (8.6%) patients with cerebrovascular disease and 287 (9.3%) patients with PAD.[31] Both treatment groups had a mean baseline LDL cholesterol level of 124 mg/dL, mean triglycerides level of 184 mg/dL, and a mean HDL level of 46 mg/dL. The mean LDL level decreased to 72 mg/dL in the atorvastatin group, while it increased to 135 mg/dL in the placebo group during follow-up. Atorvastatin significantly reduced the incidence of the primary end point when compared with placebo (14.8% vs 17.4%, RRR 84% [95% CI 70–100%], p = 0.048). The overall benefit was driven by a reduced incidence of recurrent symptomatic ischemia.[31] The reduction in the composite primary end point occurred independent of baseline LDL levels. While this study was underpowered to detect differences in the individual components of the primary end point, it did show a benefit of early therapy (randomization occurred within 24–96 hours) that was evident over 16 weeks of treatment.[31]

The Pravastatin or Atorvastatin Evaluation and Infection Therapy-Thrombolysis in Myocardial Infarction 22 (PROVE IT-TIMI 22) trial enrolled high-risk patients within 10 days of an acute coronary syndrome and randomized them to pravastatin 40 mg (moderate statin therapy) daily or atorvastatin 80 mg daily (intensive statin therapy) and followed them for an average of 24 months. The primary composite outcome measure was time to occurrence of death from any cause, MI, unstable angina, coronary revascularization, or stroke. A total of 4162 subjects were enrolled, including 241 (5.8%) patients with PAD. The LDL level decreased from 106 mg/dL to 95 mg/dL in the moderate treatment group, and from 106 mg/dL to 62 mg/dL in the intensive treatment group.[32] Atorvastatin significantly reduced the primary end point compared with pravastatin therapy (22.4% vs 26.3%, hazard rate ratio (HRR) 16% [95% CI 5–25%], $p = 0.005$). The benefit became apparent after 30 days of treatment and increased over the duration of the study.

The A to Z trial compared intensive and conservative statin therapy inpatients with ST or non-ST elevation MI with high-risk features.[33] Patients were randomized to receive simvastatin 40 mg for 30 days followed by 80 mg thereafter (intensive) or to placebo for 4 months followed by simvastatin 20 mg (conservative). The mean time from onset of symptoms to randomization was 3.7 days, and the median follow-up time was 721 days. A total of 4497 patients were randomized. The reduction in mean LDL level was 41% in the intensive group vs 27% in the conservative group at 24 months ($p < 0.001$). The primary end point of cardiovascular death, MI, readmission for acute coronary syndrome (ACS), and stroke was lower in the patients in the intensive group compared to the conservative low-dose group, but not significantly (16.7% vs 14.4%, HRR 11% [95% CI -4–24%], $p = 0.14$).[33] The event rates were lower than expected and may have limited the trial's statistical power.

Statins for peripheral arterial disease

Taken together, the above trial data demonstrate that statins reduce the incidence of cardiovascular events among those with PAD. However, few trials have been designed to specifically evaluate the effect of statins on the clinical manifestations of PAD. The Arterial Biology for the Investigation of the Treatment Effects of Reducing Cholesterol (ARBITER) and ASAP trials evaluated the progression of carotid intima media thickness (CIMT) in patients treated with atorvastatin 80 mg (intensive) vs pravastatin 40 mg or simvastatin 40 mg (conservative), respectively. CIMT is a validated surrogate for CAD and its progression can predict future cardiovascular events.[34,35] Patients in ASAP had familial hypercholesterolemia and were followed for 2 years,[36] while those in ARBITER were required to meet National Cholesterol Education Program/Adult Treatment Panel II (NCEP ATPII) criteria for pharmacological treatment and were followed for 1 year.[37] Both trials showed regression of CIMT with intensive compared with conservative therapy.

Early observational studies suggested a benign course for patients with intermittent claudication, with less than 30% of patients having progression of symptoms over 5–10 years.[38–40] However, a more recent prospective cohort study demonstrated that subjects with PAD have more substantial progression of symptoms and increasing functional decline.[41] Low ABI was associated with decreasing walking endurance after 2 years of follow-up. Furthermore, subjects with symptomatic PAD were found to have greater declines in 6-min walking tests than did matched subjects without PAD.[41]

Statins appear to play a role in improving the symptoms of PAD as well. There is an increasing body of data showing improved walking endurance in patients with intermittent claudication treated with statins.[42–44] Several recent studies evaluated the impact of simvastatin and atorvastatin on walking parameters in symptomatic patients with PAD. One study randomized patients over age 60, with intermittent claudication, mean LDL levels over 125 mg/dL, and ABI at rest less than 0.9 to simvastatin ($n = 31$) or placebo ($n = 29$). Subjects allocated to simvastatin had a significant increase in pain-free walking time at 6 months and 1 year on a standardized treadmill protocol compared to subjects treated with placebo.[45] A second study randomized patients with stable intermittent claudication without rest pain, but with evidence of PAD on ultrasound or angiography, resting ABI less than 0.9, and total serum cholesterol over 220 mg/dL[44] to simvastatin ($n = 43$) or placebo ($n = 43$). Pain-free and total walking distance was significantly improved in the simvastatin compared with placebo group after 3 months of therapy. While this study showed an improvement in the resting and post-exercise ABI, the improvement over placebo was not large enough to explain the improved walking distance.[44] The results of these studies are in line with a 4S substudy that found the risk of new or worsening intermittent claudication to be 38% lower ($p = 0.008$) in the simvastatin compared with placebo group after 5 years of follow-up.[46] Finally, one multicenter, randomized controlled trial has assessed the effect of atorvastatin on claudication symptoms.[43] A total of 364 patients with intermittent claudication and resting ABI under 0.9 were randomized to atorvastatin 10 mg, 80 mg, or placebo (data are reported on 354 patients) and patients were tested at baseline and after 12 months of therapy. The ABI was not significantly different between groups at 12 months. While there was a trend towards greater maximal walking time (MWT, in seconds) in both atorvastatin-treated groups, the difference between these groups was not statistically significant. Mean pain-free walking time (PFWT, in seconds) improved significantly more in the atorvastatin 80 mg group compared to the placebo group.[43] There was no significant difference between the atorvastatin 10 mg and placebo-treated groups. On post hoc analyses, LDL levels and smoking did not affect the response to atorvastatin.

Fibrates for atherosclerotic cardiovascular disease

Low HDL has been associated with PAD in various population studies.[7–11,18] In addition to raising HDL, fibric acid derivatives improve endothelial function,[47,48] and have anti-inflammatory effects.[49] The Veterans Affairs High-Density Lipoprotein Cholesterol Intervention Trial (VA-HIT) was designed to evaluate the effect of gemfibrozil for secondary prevention in patients with CAD because of the high prevalence of low or average LDL levels in combination with low HDL and high triglycerides among such patients. A total of 2531 patients randomized to gemfibrozil or placebo were followed for a median of 5.1 years. The primary outcome was a composite of non-fatal MI or death due to CAD. At baseline, mean HDL cholesterol was 32 mg/dL, mean LDL levels 111 mg/dL, and there was a high prevalence of diabetes (25%), hypertension (57%), and abdominal obesity.[50] After 1 year of treatment, the mean HDL level was 6% higher in the treatment compared with the placebo group, and the mean triglyceride level was 31% lower. Both differences persisted during the length of the study. There was no difference in LDL cholesterol levels.[50] Gemfibrozil significantly reduced the incidence of non-fatal MI or death due to CAD by 22% (21.7% vs 17.3, RRR 22% [95% CI 7–35%], $p = 0.006$) in the treatment group. This degree of improvement is similar to that seen in the Helsinki Heart Study, a primary prevention trial that utilized the same agent.[51,52] Finally, treatment with gemfibrozil led to non-significant reductions in the rate of confirmed stroke (6% vs 4.6%, RRR 25% [95% CI −6–47%], $p = 0.098$) and significant reductions in transient ischemic attacks (TIAs) (RRR 59%, [95% CI 33–75%], $p < 0.001$) and need for carotid endarterectomy (RRR 65% [95% CI 37–80%], $p < 0.001$).[50,53] The beneficial effects of gemfibrozil therapy were evident after 2 years of treatment, a pattern also observed in the Helsinki Heart Study.[52]

Fibrates for peripheral arterial disease

The LEADER trial enrolled 1568 patients with PAD (20% with a history of MI and 22–25% with stable angina) and randomized them to bezafibrate or placebo. The primary end point was a composite of all fatal and non-fatal coronary events, and all strokes. At baseline, the mean HDL level was 42 mg/dL. After 4.6 years of follow-up, there was an 8% increase in mean HDL level and an 8.1% decrease in LDL.[54] While there was no difference in the primary end point, there was a significant reduction in the risk of non-fatal coronary events by 40%, results that were similar to those observed in the Bezafibrate Infarction Prevention trial.[55] Additionally, improvements were noted on the Edinburgh claudication questionnaire in the benzafibrate group during the first 3 years.[54] Finally, some small angiographic studies have shown slower progression and even regression in femoral artery and coronary atherosclerosis in patients treated with fibrates, one possible mechanism for the observed symptom improvement.[47,56,57]

Nicotinic acid derivatives and atherosclerotic cardiovascular disease

The Coronary Drug Project (CDP) was a multi-arm randomized, placebo-controlled trial that enrolled men with CAD with prior MI. A total of 1103 patients were randomized to 1.8 g/day of clofibrate, 1119 patients were randomized to 3 g/day of niacin, and 2789 patients to placebo. The mean follow-up time was 6.2 years and the primary end point was total mortality.[58] The mean decreases in total cholesterol and triglycerides were 9.9% and 26%, respectively, in the niacin group, and 6.5% and 22%, respectively, in the clofibrate group.[58] There was no difference in the rate of 5-year total mortality between the treatment and placebo groups, but there was a non-significant mortality reduction in the niacin over the placebo group at the conclusion of the study. Niacin-treated subjects had a significantly lower incidence of non-fatal MI (12.2 vs 8.9%) compared to the placebo group that was evident after 2–3 years of treatment,[58] and a long-term evaluation was performed on the participants of the CDP trial 8.8 years after study termination. After 15 years of total follow-up, all-cause mortality was significantly reduced in the niacin group (58% vs 52%).[59] The difference was primarily due to a lower rate of CAD death, and was evident across most subgroups.

Nicotinic acid derivatives and peripheral arterial disease

Nicotinic acid also has benefit in patients with PAD. In a randomized trial of patients with stable claudication comparing medical therapy to usual care (dietary treatment), nicotinic acid retarded the progression of femoral artery atherosclerosis after 24 months when administered in conjunction with cholestyramine.[60] The Cholesterol Lowering Atherosclerosis Study (CLAS) was a randomized, angiographic study comparing the effects of colestipol and niacin vs diet on femoral artery atherosclerosis.[61] A total of 162 patients with coronary disease and asymptomatic PAD were randomized and followed for 24 months. Angiography showed slower progression in the proximal segments of the femoral arteries (but no difference in the other segments evaluated) in the treatment group and less progression in those patients with higher on-treatment HDL levels.[61] In another small but randomized, double-blind study, treatment with nicotinic acid led to lower cholesterol and fibrinogen levels and improved claudication symptoms.[62]

NCEP-guided care in patients with atherosclerotic vascular disease

Epidemiological studies demonstrate a log-linear relation between LDL level and risk of cardiovascular events. Secondary prevention trials show that as the LDL level is reduced, the relative risk of cardiovascular events is decreased.[63–68] Risk reductions on the order of 1% per 1 mg/dL of LDL lowering can be achieved from any given baseline LDL level.[63] Until recently, the ATPIII guidelines have recommended LDL levels of less than 100 mg/dL for high-risk patients, such as those with PAD.[64] Recent trials have provided evidence that reducing LDL levels to less than 70 mg/dL can improve cardiovascular outcomes and this target is now considered a 'therapeutic option.'

Statins and peripheral vascular interventions

Patients undergoing peripheral vascular interventions represent an important hjgh-risk cohort with severe PAD in whom secondary vascular disease prevention is likely to be particularly beneficial and cost-effective. In one study, after adjustment for demographics and comorbidities, periprocedural statin therapy was associated with a reduction in the odds of death, MI, and stroke at 6 months of 79% (95% CI 14–95%, $p = 0.03$).[69] As with patients undergoing coronary interventions, periprocedural statin therapy should be considered in all patients undergoing peripheral vascular interventions.

Statins and vascular surgery

Patients undergoing major vascular surgery also represent a cohort of patients with PAD at high risk for cardiac complications. A recently published retrospective, observational study revealed that statin therapy was associated with a lower incidence of major adverse cardiovascular events in patients undergoing aortic, carotid and lower extremity vascular surgery[70]. The odds of peri-operative death, MI, ischemia, congestive heart failure, or ventricular tachycardia were reduced by 44% when patients receiving statins were compared to patients not receiving statins during their hospitalization (95% CI 21–61%, $p = 0.0012$). This composite benefit was driven by a significant reduction in peri-operative myocardial ischemia. Further randomized, prospective studies will better define the role of statins in high risk PAD patients undergoing revascularization.

Key points

- Lipid-modifying therapy is now indicated in nearly all patients with atherosclerotic vascular disease, as multiple large secondary prevention trials have demonstrated that statins improve cardiovascular outcomes in patients with CAD and PAD.
- Statins delay disease progression and result in symptomatic improvement in patients with PAD.
- Updated NCEP ATPIII guidelines recommend a target LDL cholesterol level of <100 mg/dL with a therapeutic option of <70 mg/dL in high-risk patients such as those with PAD.
- Non-statin lipid-modifying medications such as fibrates and niacin also play a role in reducing cardiovascular outcomes, improving endothelial function, and delaying plaque progression.

References

1. Kannel WB, Castelli WP, and Gordon T. Cholesterol in the prediction of atherosclerotic disease. New perspectives based on the Framingham study. Ann Intern Med 1979;90(1):85–91.

2. Kannel WB. Range of serum cholesterol values in the population developing coronary artery disease. Am J Cardiol 1995;76(9):69C–77C.

3. Multiple Risk Factor Intervention Trial Research Group. Multiple risk factor intervention trial. Risk factor changes and mortality results. Multiple Risk Factor Intervention Trial Research Group. JAMA 1982;248(12):1465–77.

4. Castelli WP. Epidemiology of coronary heart disease: the Framingham study. Am J Med 1984;76(2A):4–12.

5. Stamler J, Wentworth D, Neaton J.D. Is relationship between serum cholesterol and risk of premature death from coronary heart disease continuous and graded? Findings in 356,222 primary screenees of the Multiple Risk Factor Intervention Trial (MRFIT). JAMA 1986;256(20):2823–8.

6. Murabito JM, D'Agostino RB, Silbershatz H, Wilson WF. Intermittent claudication. A risk profile from The Framingham Heart Study. Circulation 1997;96(1):44–9.

7. Murabito JM, Evans JC, Nieto K, et al. Prevalence and clinical correlates of peripheral arterial disease in the Framingham Offspring Study. Am Heart J 2002;143(6):961–5.

8. Newman AB, Siscovick DS, Manolio TA, et al. Ankle-arm index as a marker of atherosclerosis in the Cardiovascular Health Study. Cardiovascular Heart Study (CHS) Collaborative Research Group. Circulation 1993;88(3):837–45.

9. Fabsitz RR, Sidawy AN, Go O, et al. Prevalence of peripheral arterial disease and associated risk factors in American Indians: the Strong Heart Study. Am J Epidemiol 1999;149(4):330–8.

10. Curb J.D, Masaki K, Rodriguez BL, et al. Peripheral artery disease and cardiovascular risk factors in the elderly. The Honolulu Heart Program. Arterioscler Thromb Vasc Biol 1996;16(12):1495–500.

11. Fowkes FG, Housley E, Riemersma RA, et al. Smoking, lipids, glucose intolerance, and blood pressure as risk factors for peripheral atherosclerosis compared with ischemic heart disease in the Edinburgh Artery Study. Am J Epidemiol 1992;135(4):331–40.

12. Buchwald H, Vasco RL, Matts JP, et al. Effect of partial ileal bypass surgery on mortality and morbidity from coronary heart disease in patients with hypercholesterolemia. Report of the Program on the Surgical Control of the Hyperlipidemias (POSCH). N Engl J Med 1990;323(14):946–55.

13. Heart Protection Study Collaboration Group. MRC/BHF Heart Protection Study of cholesterol lowering with simvastatin in 20,536 high-risk individuals: a randomised placebo-controlled trial. Lancet 2002;360(9326):7–22.

14. Prevention of cardiovascular events and death with pravastatin in patients with coronary heart disease and a broad range of initial cholesterol levels. The Long-Term Intervention with Pravastatin in Ischaemic Disease (LIPID) Study Group. N Engl J Med 1998;339(19):1349–57.

15. Scandinavian Simvastatin Survival Study Group. Randomised trial of cholesterol lowering in 4444 patients with coronary heart disease: the Scandinavian Simvastatin Survival Study (4S). Lancet 1994;344(8934):1383–9.

16. The LIPID Study Group. Long-term effectiveness and safety of pravastatin in 9014 patients with coronary heart disease and average cholesterol concentrations: the LIPID trial follow-up. Lancet 2002;359(9315):1379–87.

17. Sacks FM, Pfeffer MA, Moye LA, et al. The effect of pravastatin on coronary events after myocardial infarction in patients with average cholesterol levels. Cholesterol and Recurrent Events Trial investigators. N Engl J Med 1996;335(14):1001–9.

18. Rubins HB, Robins SJ, Collins D, et al. Distribution of lipids in 8,500 men with coronary artery disease. Department of Veterans Affairs HDL Intervention Trial Study Group. Am J Cardiol 1995;75(17):1196–201.

19. Wilt TJ, Davis BR, Meyers DG, Rouleau JL, Sacks FM. Prevalence and correlates of symptomatic peripheral atherosclerosis in individuals with coronary heart disease and cholesterol levels less than 240 mg/dL: baseline results from the Cholesterol and Recurrent Events (CARE) Study. Angiology 1996;47(6):533–41.

20. Arday DR, Fleming BB, Keller DK, et al. Variation in diabetes care among states: do patient characteristics matter? Diabetes Care 2002;25(12):2230–7.

21. Rowland Yeo K, Yeo WW. Lipid lowering in patients with diabetes mellitus: what coronary heart disease risk threshold should be used? Heart 2002;87(5):423–7.

22. Thomason MJ, Colhoun HM, Livingstone SJ, et al. Baseline characteristics in the Collaborative AtoRvastatin Diabetes Study (CARDS) in patients with Type 2 diabetes. Diabet Med 2004;21(8):901–5.

23. Collins R, Armitage J, Parish S, et al. MRC/BHF Heart Protection Study of cholesterol-lowering with simvastatin in 5963 people with diabetes: a randomised placebo-controlled trial. Lancet 2003;361(9374):2005–16.

24. Downs JR, Clearfield M, Weis S, et al. Primary prevention of acute coronary events with lovastatin in men and women with average cholesterol levels: results of AFCAPS/TexCAPS. Air Force/Texas Coronary Atherosclerosis Prevention Study. JAMA 1998;279(20):1615–22.

25. White HD, Simes RJ, Anderson NE, et al. Pravastatin therapy and the risk of stroke. N Engl J Med 2000;343(5):317–26.

26. Plehn JF, Davis BR, Sacks FM, et al. Reduction of stroke incidence after myocardial infarction with pravastatin: the Cholesterol and Recurrent Events (CARE) study. The Care Investigators. Circulation 1999;99(2):216–23.

27. Collins R, Armitage J, Parish S, et al. Effects of cholesterol-lowering with simvastatin on stroke and other major vascular events in 20536 people with cerebrovascular disease or other high-risk conditions. Lancet 2004;363(9411):757–67.

28. Shepherd J, Blauw GJ, Murphy MB, et al. Pravastatin in elderly individuals at risk of vascular disease (PROSPER): a randomised controlled trial Lancet, 2002;360(9346):1623–30.

29. Schillinger M, Exner M, Mlekusch W, et al. Statin therapy improves cardiovascular outcome of patients with peripheral artery disease. Eur Heart J 2004;25(9):742–8.

30. Aronow HD, Topol EJ, Roe MT, et al. Effect of lipid-lowering therapy on early mortality after acute coronary syndromes: an observational study. Lancet 2001;357(9262):1063–8.

31. Schwartz GG, Olsson AG, Ezekowitz MD, et al. Effects of atorvastatin on early recurrent ischemic events in acute coronary syndromes: the MIRACL study: a randomized controlled trial. JAMA 2001;285(13):1711–18.

32. Cannon CP, Braunwald E, McCabe CH, et al. Intensive versus moderate lipid lowering with statins after acute coronary syndromes. N Engl J Med 2004;350(15):1495–504.

33. de Lemos JA, Blazing MA, Wiviott SD, et al. Early intensive vs a delayed conservative simvastatin strategy in patients with acute coronary syndromes: phase Z of the A to Z trial. JAMA 2004;292(11):1307–16.

34. Hodis HN, Mack WJ, LaBree L, et al. The role of carotid arterial intima-media thickness in predicting clinical coronary events. Ann Intern Med 1998;128(4):262–9.

35. Salonen R, Nyyssonen K, Porkkala E, et al. Kuopio Atherosclerosis Prevention Study (KAPS). A population-based primary preventive trial of the effect of LDL lowering on atherosclerotic progression in carotid and femoral arteries. Circulation 1995;92(7):1758–64.

36. Smilde TJ, van Wissen S, Wollersheim H, et al. Effect of aggressive versus conventional lipid lowering on atherosclerosis progression in familial hypercholesterolaemia (ASAP): a prospective, randomised, double-blind trial. Lancet 2001;357(9256):577–81.

37. Taylor AJ, Kent SM, Flaherty PJ, et al. ARBITER: Arterial Biology for the Investigation of the Treatment Effects of Reducing Cholesterol: a randomized trial comparing the effects of atorvastatin and pravastatin on carotid intima medial thickness. Circulation 2002;106(16):2055–60.

38. Imparato AM, Kim GE, Davidson T, Crowley JG. Intermittent claudication: its natural course. Surgery 1975;78(6):795–9.

39. McAllister FF. The fate of patients with intermittent claudication managed nonoperatively. Am J Surg 1976;132(5):593–5.

40. Boyd AM. The natural course of arteriosclerosis of the lower extremities. Proc R Soc Med 1962;55:591–3.

41. McDermott MM, Liu K, Greenland P, et al. Functional decline in peripheral arterial disease: associations with the ankle brachial index and leg symptoms. JAMA 2004;292(4):453–61.

42. McDermott MM, Guralnik JM, Greenland P, et al. Statin use and leg functioning in patients with and without lower-extremity peripheral arterial disease. Circulation 2003;107(5):757–61.

43. Mohler ER 3rd, Hiatt WR, Creager MA. Cholesterol reduction with atorvastatin improves walking distance in patients with peripheral arterial disease. Circulation 2003;108(12):1481–6.

44. Mondillo S, Ballo P, Barbati R, et al. Effects of simvastatin on walking performance and symptoms of intermittent claudication in hypercholesterolemic patients with peripheral vascular disease. Am J Med 2003;114(5):359–64.

45. Aronow WS, Nayak D, Woodworth S, Ahn C. Effect of simvastatin versus placebo on treadmill exercise time until the onset of intermittent claudication in older patients with peripheral arterial disease at six months and at one year after treatment. Am J Cardiol 2003;92(6):711–12.

46. Pedersen TR, Kjekshus J, Pyorala K et al. Effect of simvastatin on ischemic signs and symptoms in the Scandinavian simvastatin survival study (4S). Am J Cardiol 1998;81(3):333–5.

47. Frick MH, Syvanne M, Nieminen MS, et al. Prevention of the angiographic progression of coronary and vein-graft atherosclerosis by gemfibrozil after coronary bypass surgery in men with low levels of HDL cholesterol. Lopid Coronary Angiography Trial (LOCAT) Study Group. Circulation 1997; 96(7):2137–43.

48. Seiler C, Suter TM, Hess OM. Exercise-induced vasomotion of angiographically normal and stenotic coronary arteries improves after cholesterol-lowering drug therapy with bezafibrate. J Am Coll Cardiol 1995;26(7):1615–22.

49. Madej A, Okopien B, Kowalski J, et al. Effects of fenofibrate on plasma cytokine concentrations in patients with atherosclerosis and hyperlipoproteinemia IIb. Int J Clin Pharmacol Ther 1998;36(6):345–9.

50. Rubins HB, Robins SJ, Collins D, et al. Gemfibrozil for the secondary prevention of coronary heart disease in men with low levels of high-density lipoprotein cholesterol. Veterans Affairs High-Density Lipoprotein Cholesterol Intervention Trial Study Group. N Engl J Med 1999;341(6):410–18.

51. Manninen V, Elo MO, Frick MH, et al. Lipid alterations and decline in the incidence of coronary heart disease in the Helsinki Heart Study. JAMA 1988;260(5):641–51.

52. Frick MH, Elo O, Haapa K, et al. Helsinki Heart Study: primary-prevention trial with gemfibrozil in middle-aged men with dyslipidemia. Safety of treatment, changes in risk factors, and incidence of coronary heart disease. N Engl J Med 1987;317(20):1237–45.

53. Bloomfield Rubins H, Davenport J, Babikian V, et al. Reduction in stroke with gemfibrozil in men with coronary heart disease and low HDL cholesterol: The Veterans Affairs HDL Intervention Trial (VA-HIT). Circulation 2001;103(23):2828–33.

54. Meade T, Zuhrie R, Cook C, Cooper J. Bezafibrate in men with lower extremity arterial disease: randomised controlled trial. BMJ 2002;325(7373):1139.

55. The BIP Study Group. Secondary prevention by raising HDL cholesterol and reducing triglycerides in patients with coronary artery disease: the Bezafibrate Infarction Prevention (BIP) study. Circulation 2000;102(1):21–7.

56. Barndt R Jr, Crawford DW. A new three-dimensional postmortem method to study the topography of atherosclerosis using profilometry. Atherosclerosis 1977;27(2):121–8.

57. Diabetes Atherosclerosis Intervention Study Investigators. Effect of fenofibrate on progression of coronary-artery disease in type 2 diabetes: the Diabetes Atherosclerosis Intervention Study, a randomised study. Lancet 2001;357(9260):905–10.

58. Clofibrate and niacin in coronary heart disease. JAMA 1975;231(4):360–81.

59. Canner PL, Berge KG, Wenger NK, et al. Fifteen year mortality in Coronary Drug Project patients: long-term benefit with niacin. J Am Coll Cardiol 1986;8(6):1245–55.

60. Duffield RG, Lewis B, Miller NE, et al. Treatment of hyperlipidaemia retards progression of symptomatic femoral atherosclerosis. A randomised controlled trial. Lancet 1983;2(8351):639–42.

61. Blankenhorn DH, Azen SP, Crawford DW, et al. Effects of colestipol-niacin therapy on human femoral atherosclerosis. Circulation 1991;83(2):438–47.

62. Davis E, Rozov H. Xanthinol nicotinate in peripheral vascular disease. Practitioner 1975;215(1290):793–8.

63. Grundy SM, Cleeman JI, Merz CN, et al. Implications of recent clinical trials for the National Cholesterol Education Program Adult Treatment Panel III guidelines. Arterioscler Thromb Vasc Biol 2004;24(8):149–61.

64. Expert Panel on Detection, Evaluation, and Treatment of High Blood Cholesterol in Adults. Executive Summary of The Third Report of The National Cholesterol Education Program (NCEP) Expert Panel on Detection, Evaluation, and Treatment of High Blood Cholesterol In Adults (Adult Treatment Panel III). JAMA 2001;285(19):2486–97.

65. Grundy SM, Cleeman JI, Merz CN, et al. Implications of recent clinical trials for the National Cholesterol Education Program Adult Treatment Panel III guidelines. Circulation 2004;110(2):227–39.

66. Furberg CD, Adams HP Jr, Applegate WB, et al. Effect of lovastatin on early carotid atherosclerosis and cardiovascular events. Asymptomatic Carotid Artery Progression Study (ACAPS) Research Group. Circulation 1994;90(4):1679–87.

67. Nissen SE, Tuzcu EM, Schoenhagen P, et al. Effect of intensive compared with moderate lipid-lowering therapy on progression of coronary atherosclerosis: a randomized controlled trial. JAMA 2004;291(9):1071–80.

68. Ost CR, Stenson S. Regression of peripheral atherosclerosis during therapy with high doses of nicotinic acid. Scand J Clin Lab Invest Suppl 1967;99:241–5.

69. Dey S, Mukherjee D. Clinical perspectives on the role of anti-platelet and statin therapy in patients with vascular diseases. Curr Vasc Pharmacol 2003;1(3):329–33.

70. O'Neil-Callahan K, Katzimaglis G, Tepper MR, et al. Statins decrease perioperative cardiac complications in patients undergoing noncardiac vascular surgery. J Am Coll Cardiol 2005;45:336–42.

5. RENIN–ANGIOTENSIN–ALDOSTERONE SYSTEM (RAAS) BLOCKADE IN PERIPHERAL ARTERIAL DISEASES

Bertram Pitt, Debabrata Mukherjee and Sanjay Rajagopalan

Atherosclerosis remains the most common cause of peripheral arterial disease (PAD), and pharmacological agents that alter the central process of atherosclerosis may have the potential to alter the natural history of PAD. There is increasing evidence that the renin–angiotensin–aldosterone system (RAAS) is a significant mediator of the atherosclerotic disease process (Fig. 5.1) and that treatment with angiotensin-converting enzyme (ACE) inhibitors, angiotensin receptor blockers (ARBs) or aldosterone blockers (ABs) may be associated with vasculoprotective effects that are independent of the antihypertensive and/or diuretic properties of these agents. Several studies have shown that ACE inhibitors directly inhibit the atherosclerotic process and may improve vascular endothelial function. In patients with PAD, ACE inhibitors have been shown to improve peripheral circulation, as measured by peripheral

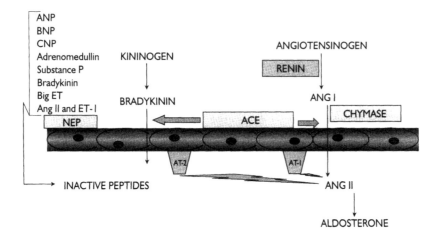

Figure 5.1 Components of the renin–angiotensin–aldosterone neutral endopeptidase (NEP) pathway. ACE = angiotensin-converting enzyme; Ang II = angiotensin II; ET = endothelin; ANP = atrial natriuretic peptide; BNP = brain natriuretic peptide; CNP = C-type natriuretic peptide; AT-1 = angiotensin type 1 receptor; AT-2 = angiotensin type 2 receptor.

arterial blood pressure and by increases in peripheral blood flow. Preliminary evidence suggests that ACE inhibitors might also improve clinical symptoms in patients with PAD. Recent evidence has confirmed that ACE inhibition is associated with a decrease in morbidity and mortality in patients with arterial disease without left ventricular dysfunction; this benefit was at least as great if not greater for the subset of patients with PAD. Overall, the data support a significant role for the RAAS in the pathogenesis of all atherosclerotic diseases, including PAD and cerebrovascular diseases, and suggest that the benefit is independent of the blood pressure lowering properties of these agents. These and other studies suggest that ACE/ARB inhibitor therapy should be considered in the routine management of individuals with PAD, regardless of whether they have hypertension or left ventricular dysfunction.[1]

Angiotensin-converting enzyme inhibitors

Blockade of the RAAS by ACE inhibitors (Fig. 5.2) slows progression of atherosclerosis in animal models, decreases morbidity and mortality in patients with heart failure, reduces rates of cardiovascular morbidity and mortality in

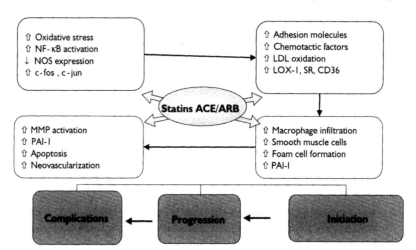

Figure 5.2 *Common pathways relevant in initiation, progression, and complications of atherosclerosis that are prevented by statins, angiotensin-converting enzyme inhibitors (ACEI) and angiotensin receptor blockers (ARBs). NF-κB = nuclear factor-κB; c-fos and c-jun are early response transcription factors that are activated by a number of mitogenic stimuli important in response to injury; LDL = low-density lipoproteins; LOX-1 = lectin-like oxidized low-density lipoprotein receptor; SR = scavenger receptor (class A); CD36 = scavenger receptor class B type I (SR-BI); MMP = matrix metalloproteinase; PAI-1 = plasminogen activator inhibitor-1; NOS, nitric oxide synthase.*

high-risk patients (e.g. those with diabetes), controls blood pressure, and delays the progression of renal failure.[2] In addition, it has been shown to inhibit cellular proliferation, decrease apoptosis, and inhibit fibrosis in the vasculature, heart, and kidneys.

Ostergren et al assessed the prognostic importance of PAD as evaluated by ankle–brachial index (ABI), and the impact of ramipril on the prevention of major cardiovascular events in PAD patients included in the Heart Outcomes Prevention Evaluation (HOPE) study.[3] In this study, patients were randomized to treatment with ramipril or placebo and followed for 4.5 years. The ABI was measured, mainly by digital palpation of the foot pulse, at baseline in 8986 patients. The ABI was subnormal (≤0.9) in 3099 patients and normal in 5887 patients. A low ABI was a strong predictor of morbidity and mortality during the follow-up, even in patients with no clinical symptoms of PAD ($n = 6769$). Ramipril significantly improved clinical outcomes in patients with a clinical history of PAD as well as in patients with subclinical PAD.[3] The study suggested that the ABI, even if measured simply by palpation of the foot arteries, is a strong predictor for future cardiovascular events and for all-cause mortality and that the ACE inhibitor ramipril prevented major cardiovascular events in patients with clinical as well as subclinical PAD.

Bosch et al determined the effect of ramipril on the secondary prevention of stroke in 9297 patients with vascular disease or diabetes plus an additional risk factor, followed for 4.5 years as part of the same HOPE study.[4] Stroke, confirmed by computed tomography (CT) or magnetic resonance imaging (MRI) when available, transient ischemic attack, and cognitive function were the primary outcomes studied for this analysis. Blood pressure was recorded at entry to the study, after 2 years, and at the end of the study. Overall, reduction in blood pressure was modest (3.8 mmHg systolic and 2.8 mmHg diastolic) with ramipril. However, the relative risk of any stroke was reduced by 32% (156 vs 226) in the ramipril group compared with the placebo group, and the relative risk of fatal stroke was reduced by 61% (17 vs 44). Benefits were consistent across baseline blood pressures, drugs used, and subgroups, defined by the presence or absence of previous stroke, coronary artery disease, peripheral arterial disease, diabetes, or hypertension. Significantly fewer patients on ramipril had cognitive or functional impairment. The study showed that ramipril reduces the incidence of stroke in patients at high risk, despite a modest reduction in blood pressure. In the Study to Evaluate Carotid Ultrasound Changes in Patients Treated With Ramipril and Vitamin E (SECURE) substudy, which looked at the progression of atherosclerosis as evaluated by B-mode carotid ultrasound, ramipril significantly slowed the progression of atherosclerosis ($p = 0.033$).[5]

The Perindopril Protection Against Recurrent Stroke Study (PROGRESS) investigated the efficacy of the ACE inhibitor perindopril alone and in combination with the diuretic indapamide in reducing the risk of stroke in 6105 hypertensive and nonhypertensive patients with a history of stroke or transient ischemic attack.[6] In the study, patients were randomly assigned to receive either active treatment ($n = 3051$) or placebo ($n = 3054$). Patients in the active treatment group received 4 mg of perindopril daily; indapamide therapy was added at the discretion of the treating physician. Over the 4-year follow-up period, active therapy reduced blood pressure by 9/4 mmHg and reduced the risk of stroke by 28% and total major vascular events by 26%. The risk reduction in stroke was similar between hypertensive and nonhypertensive patients. Those patients who received perindopril plus indapamide had a 12/5 mmHg drop in blood pressure and a 43% reduction in the risk of stroke.

The results from the Second Australian National Blood Pressure Study suggested that ACE inhibition may be preferable to diuretic use for cardiovascular risk reduction, especially in older male patients. Subjects with hypertension and aged 65–84 years were prospectively studied in this randomized open-label trial with blinded assessment of end points. The 6083 participants received either an ACE inhibitor (enalapril) or a diuretic (hydrochlorothiazide) and were observed for a median of 4.1 years. Blood pressure reduction (26/12 mmHg) was similar between groups, but the risk of all cardiovascular events or death from any cause was 11% lower with the ACE inhibitor than with the diuretic ($p = 0.05$), which indicated a benefit in cardiovascular risk reduction beyond that of blood pressure reduction.[7] The efficacy of perindopril in reduction of cardiovascular events among patients with stable coronary artery disease (EUROPA) trial demonstrated that among patients with stable coronary heart disease without apparent heart failure, perindopril significantly improves clinical outcome.[8] The study suggested that treatment with perindopril, on top of other preventive medications, should be considered in all patients with vascular disease with or without heart failure.[8]

Angiotensin receptor blockers

The ARBs act by selectively binding to and blocking the angiotensin II type 1 (AT_1) receptor. The deleterious responses to angiotensin II, the main effector peptide of the RAAS, are mediated through the AT_1 receptor. Such responses include vasoconstriction, aldosterone and vasopressin secretion, sympathetic nervous system activation, renal tubular sodium reabsorption, and decreased renal blood flow. Angiotensin II has been shown to cause an increase in vascular NADPH oxidase activity, an increase in the production of reactive oxygen species (ROS), vascular inflammation, and the progression of atherosclerosis (see Fig. 5.2). Angiotensin II also activates the LOX-1 receptors responsible for the oxidation of LDL-cholesterol and therefore causes a further increase in ROS. Angiotensin II has also been shown to be associated with plaque growth, which is an important factor in the progression of atherosclerosis, as well as to enhance the tendency for thrombosis and to impair fibrinolysis. These effects can be prevented by either the administration of an ACE inhibitor and or an ARB.

Among ARBs, losartan is indicated for reducing the risk of stroke in patients with hypertension and left ventricular hypertrophy, irbesartan and losartan are indicated for the treatment of diabetic nephropathy in patients with type 2 diabetes and hypertension, and valsartan is indicated for the treatment of heart failure (New York Heart Association class II-IV) in patients intolerant of ACE inhibitors and hypertension. The Valsartan in Acute Myocardial Infarction (VALIANT) trial demonstrated that valsartan was as effective as captopril in patients who are at high risk for cardiovascular events after myocardial infarction, but combining valsartan with captopril increased the rate of adverse events without improving survival.[9] However, in the Candesartan in Heart failure: Assessment of Reduction in Mortality and morbidity (CHARM)-Added trial, the addition of candesartan to an ACE inhibitor and other treatment led to a further clinically important reduction in relevant cardiovascular events.[10] Inhibition of RAAS may also exert an antidiabetic effect; thus, prospective studies involving ARBs, such as the Nateglinide and Valsartan in Impaired Glucose Tolerance Outcomes Research (NAVIGATOR) trial are under way to explore this observation objectively. Taken together, these clinical findings suggest that RAAS blockade by ARBs has widespread protective effects on the vasculature, provided that blood pressure is also adequately controlled. On the basis of this premise, it is likely that indications for ARBs will continue to expand further in the years to come.

Aldosterone blockers

Since angiotensin II is an important stimulus for the production of aldosterone from the adrenal gland, one might conclude that there would be little if any added benefit of an aldosterone blocker (AB) in a patient treated with an ACE inhibitor and/or ARB for vascular disease. However, angiotensin II, while an important stimulus for the production of aldosterone, is not the only one. For example, potassium is also an important stimulus for the production of aldosterone, and aldosterone can be produced in the angiotensin knockout mouse in which there is no angiotensin II.

There is increasing evidence that, despite the use of an ACE inhibitor and an ARB, while aldosterone production can be transiently suppressed it cannot be suppressed over the long term (aldosterone escape). For example, the

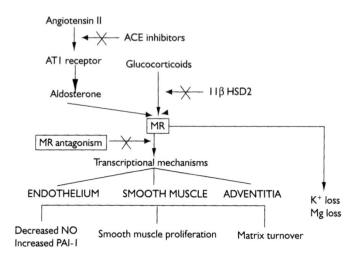

Figure 5.3 *Adverse effects of activation of the mineralocorticoid receptor (MR) and the benefits of antagonizing it. AT1 = angiotensin type 1 receptor; 11β HSD 2 = 11β-hydroxysteroid dehydrogenase type 2, an enzyme that is tightly coupled to MR, at least in the kidney and which metabolizes cortisol to cortisone, preventing the former from occupying MR; NO = nitric oxide; PAI–1 = plasminogen activator inhibitor–1.*

continuation of an ACE inhibitor and an ARB has been shown to transiently suppress aldosterone at 17 weeks but by 43 weeks aldosterone levels typically rise above control.[11] Thus, despite effective doses of an ACE inhibitor and also an ARB, aldosterone production may not be suppressed and may be potentially available to stimulate the mineralocorticoid receptor (MR) (Fig. 5.3). These receptors are classically found in the distal renal tubule and are responsible for sodium retention and potassium loss when activated by aldosterone. MR, however, are present not only in the renal tubule but also in the endothelium, myocardium, and brain. They have been shown to have important effects on vascular function, inflammation apoptosis, collagen formation, hypertrophy, collagen formation, hypertrophy and nervous system regulation and central sympathetic nervous system activation, platelet activation, and fibrinolysis. MR, while typically activated by aldosterone, can also be activated by cortisol.

Further evidence for an effect on AB in vascular disease comes from studies in the APO-1 knockout mouse. Angiotensin II has been shown to increase the atherosclerotic lesion area in this model, which can be prevented by an ARB. The atherosclerotic lesion area, however, could also be reduced by an AB, suggesting that the effect of angiotensin II in the model was in large part mediated by activation of the MR. However, while both an ARB and an AB appear similarly effective, the fact that angiotensin II inhibition or blockade may not suppress aldosterone over the long term (aldosterone escape) suggests that an ACE inhibitor and/or an ARB alone may be suboptimal to inhibit the progression of vascular disease. This concept is supported by further studies in the APO-1 knockout mouse in which aldosterone has been shown to increase LDL cholesterol oxidation and atherosclerotic lesion area. The most effective strategy to reduce atherosclerotic lesion area in the model was the combination of an AB and an ACE inhibitor over an ARB only.

Clinical implications

ACE inhibitors and ARBs effectively interfere with the renin–angiotensin system and exert various beneficial actions on cardiac and vascular structure and function, beyond their blood pressure-lowering effects. Randomized, controlled clinical trials have shown that ACE inhibitors and ARBs improve endothelial function, cardiac and vascular remodeling, retard the anatomic progression of atherosclerosis, and reduce the risk of myocardial infarction, stroke, and cardiovascular death. Therefore, these agents are recommended in the treatment of a wide range of patients at risk for adverse cardiovascular outcomes, including those with coronary disease, prior stroke, peripheral arterial disease, high-risk diabetes, hypertension, and heart failure. ARBs are effective blood pressure-lowering and renoprotective agents and can be used in heart failure in patients who do not tolerate ACE inhibitors.[12] The role of ARBs in the prevention of atherosclerosis and its sequelae is currently under active investigation. The use of combined ACE inhibitor plus ARB therapy offers theoretical advantages over the use of each of these agents alone and is also under investigation. The dosages of several commonly used ACE inhibitors, ARBs, and aldosterone blockers are listed in Table 5.1.

The HOPE[13] and the EUROPA[8] trials demonstrated the effectiveness of ACE inhibitors in reducing cardiovascular mortality, non-fatal myocardial infarction, and non-fatal stroke in patients with high-risk vascular disease including those with peripheral vascular disease, without evidence of systolic left ventricular dysfunction (SLVD) or evidence of heart failure. ACE inhibitors have been shown to slow the progression of atherosclerosis both experimentally and in patients with vascular disease, as evidenced by a decrease in carotid intimal media thickness (CIMT) in comparison to placebo. ACE inhibitors and/or ARBs have been shown to affect a number of important pathophysiological processes associated with the progression of atherosclerosis, plaque growth, thrombosis, and fibrinolysis. These mechanisms point to the important role for the RAAS in the pathophysiology of vascular disease and ACE inhibitor and/or ARBs in preventing the progression of vascular disease

Table 5.1 Dosages of commonly used ACE inhibitors, ARBs, and aldosterone blockers

Drug	Dosage
Commonly used angiotensin-converting enzyme inhibitors	
Captopril	Start at 6.25 mg orally twice or three times daily; maximum 150 mg/day
Enalapril	Start at 2.5 mg orally once a day or divided twice daily; maximum 40 mg/day
Lisinopril	Start at 10 mg orally once daily; maximum 80 mg/day
Benazepril	Start 10 mg orally once daily; maximum 80 mg per day
Fosinopril	Start at 10 mg orally once a day; maximum 80 mg orally once daily
Quinapril	Start at 10 mg orally once daily or divided twice daily; maximum 80 mg/day
Ramipril	Start at 2.5 mg orally once daily; maximum 20 mg/day
Perindopril	Start at 4 mg orally once daily; maximum 16 mg/day
Commonly used angiotension II receptor blockers	
Losartan	Start 50 mg orally once daily; maximum 100 mg/day given
Candesartan	Start 16 mg orally once a day; maximum 32 mg/day
Irbesartan	Start 75 mg orally once daily; maximum 300 mg/day
Valsartan	Start 80 mg orally once daily; maximum 320 mg/day
Telmisartan	Start at 40 mg orally once daily; maximum 80 mg/day
Aldosterone blockers	
Spironolactone	Start 50 mg orally once daily; maximum 100 mg/day given
Epleronone	Start 25 mg orally once daily; maximum 400 mg/day

and its clinical consequences. Whereas the role of angiotensin II in the pathophysiology of vascular disease is well recognized, the role of aldosterone is less clear. There are, however, a number of clues suggesting that aldosterone may also play an important pathophysiological role and that ABs may add to the efficacy of ACE inhibitor and/or ARBs in preventing the progression of vascular disease and its consequences.

Conclusions

The mechanisms and findings outlined above provide a basis for the hypothesis that blockade of the RAAS, using ACE inhibitors, ARBs, and aldosterone antagonists, will play an important role in the prevention of vascular disease and its clinical sequence. It should, however, be emphasized that well-documented prospective randomized studies will be necessary to confirm the hypothesis that AB will provide significant benefit to patients with vascular disease without left ventricular dysfunction above that provided by an ACE inhibitor and/or an ARB alone. Given this caveat, the opportunity exists for further improvement in the outcome of patients with vascular disease and in particular high-risk patients with peripheral vascular disease for blockade of the RAAS when added to other effective current therapies, including a statin and effective antiplatelet therapy.[14]

Key points

- There is increasing evidence that the RAAS is a significant mediator of the atherosclerotic disease process and that treatment with ACE inhibitors or ARBs may be associated with vasculoprotective effects independent of the antihypertensive properties of these agents.
- Several studies have shown that ACE inhibitors directly inhibit the atherosclerotic process and improve vascular endothelial function.
- ACE inhibitor/ARB therapy should be considered in the routine management of individuals with PAD, regardless of whether they have hypertension or left ventricular dysfunction.
- Aldosterone blocking agents may add to the efficacy of ACE inhibitors and/or ARBs in preventing the progression of vascular disease and its consequences.

References

1. Hirsch AT, Duprez D. The potential role of angiotensin-converting enzyme inhibition in peripheral arterial disease. Vasc Med 2003;8:273–8.

2. Burnier M. Angiotensin II type 1 receptor blockers. Circulation 2001;103:904–12.

3. Ostergren J, Sleight P, Dagenais G, et al. Impact of ramipril in patients with evidence of clinical or subclinical peripheral arterial disease. Eur Heart J 2004;25:17–24.

4. Bosch J, Yusuf S, Pogue J, et al. Use of ramipril in preventing stroke: double blind randomised trial. BMJ 2002;324:699–702.

5. Lonn E, Yusuf S, Dzavik V, et al. Effects of ramipril and vitamin E on atherosclerosis: the study to evaluate carotid ultrasound changes in patients treated with ramipril and vitamin E (SECURE). Circulation 2001;103:919–25.

6. Randomised trial of a perindopril-based blood-pressure-lowering regimen among 6,105 individuals with previous stroke or transient ischaemic attack. Lancet 2001;358:1033–41.

7. Wing LM, Reid CM, Ryan P, et al. A comparison of outcomes with angiotensin-converting–enzyme inhibitors and diuretics for hypertension in the elderly. N Engl J Med 2003;348:583–92.

8. Fox KM. Efficacy of perindopril in reduction of cardiovascular events among patients with stable coronary artery disease: randomised, double-blind, placebo-controlled, multicentre trial (the EUROPA study). Lancet 2003;362:782–8.

9. Pfeffer MA, McMurray JJ, Velazquez EJ, et al. Valsartan, captopril, or both in myocardial infarction complicated by heart failure, left ventricular dysfunction, or both. N Engl J Med 2003;349:1893–906.

10. McMurray JJ, Ostergren J, Swedberg K, et al. Effects of candesartan in patients with chronic heart failure and reduced left-ventricular systolic function taking angiotensin-converting-enzyme inhibitors: the CHARM-Added trial. Lancet 2003;362:767–71.

11. Pitt B. Effect of aldosterone blockade in patients with systolic left ventricular dysfunction: implications of the RALES and EPHESUS studies. Mol Cell Endocrinol 2004;217:53–8.

12. Lonn E. Angiotensin-converting enzyme inhibitors and angiotensin receptor blockers in atherosclerosis. Curr Atheroscler Rep 2002;4:363–72.

13. Yusuf S, Sleight P, Pogue J, et al. Effects of an angiotensin-converting-enzyme inhibitor, ramipril, on cardiovascular events in high-risk patients. The Heart Outcomes Prevention Evaluation Study Investigators. N Engl J Med 2000;342:145–53.

14. Mukherjee D, Lingam P, Chetcuti S, et al. Missed opportunities to treat atherosclerosis in patients undergoing peripheral vascular interventions: insights from the University of Michigan Peripheral Vascular Disease Quality Improvement Initiative (PVD-QI2). Circulation 2002;106:1909–12.

6. BETA-BLOCKERS IN PERIPHERAL ARTERIAL DISEASE

Joel Reginelli and Stanley J Chetcuti

Beta-blockers produce a competitive and reversible antagonism of the effects of ß-adrenergic stimulation on the body. They may have different selectivity to the β_1- and β_2-adrenergic receptors and are thus classified as (a) non-selective, and as (b) selective blockers with higher affinity for the β_1- than the β_2-receptors.[1] Selectivity may, however, be overwhelmed at higher doses. Several of the ß-adrenergic receptor antagonists may also demonstrate peripheral vasodilator activity mediated via α_1-adrenoreceptor blockade (e.g. carvedilol and labetalol). Beta-blockers play a major role in the treatment of cardiovascular disease and for many years have been used for the treatment of hypertension, ischemic heart disease, ventricular arrhythmias, hypertrophic cardiomyopathies, and, more recently, for the treatment of chronic heart failure. The theoretical concern of unopposed α_1-receptor stimulation in the presence of ß-adrenergic receptor antagonists has led to the underutilization of these drugs in patients with peripheral arterial disease (PAD).

Atherosclerosis is a systemic disease that concomitantly affects multiple vascular beds to varying degrees,[2] thus manifesting in a variety of ways. PAD, as one of these manifestations, should not be considered in isolation but within the gamut of a diffuse condition with widespread effects. It has been well described that patients with PAD are at greater risk for stroke or myocardial infarction than limb amputation. In one study of patients with PAD, the 5-year mortality rate was 30%, of which 75% of deaths were due to cardiovascular events. These rates are greater than the long-term rate for major amputation, estimated to occur in less than 4% of this patient population.[3] Several studies have demonstrated that the presence of lower extremity peripheral arterial disease is associated with significantly elevated risk for future cardiac events and mortality.[4–7]

A number of large clinical trials have demonstrated that ß-adrenergic receptor antagonist administration following myocardial infarction is associated with significant reductions in early and late mortality.[8–10] Unfortunately, physicians still prescribe ß-receptor antagonists for less than one-third[11] and cardiologists less than one-half of patients with myocardial infarction.[12] Comorbid conditions such as older age, diminished left ventricular function, transient heart failure, and diabetes and peripheral arterial disease may be the trigger for the underutilization of this class of drugs.[13] Narins et al recently demonstrated that only about half of the myocardial infarction survivors with symptomatic peripheral arterial disease receive ß-blocker therapy 2 months following their index event, a proportion that was significantly lower than that observed among patients without claudication.[14] The reasons for this underutilization of ß-blocker therapy among postinfarction patients with claudication are probably multifactorial. Because of the concern that ß-blocking agents may further reduce blood flow through diseased peripheral arteries, the presence of claudication has been viewed as a relative contraindication for this form of therapy.[15] There is not much objective evidence to substantiate this contention. In fact, skin microcirculation, as assessed with three noninvasive techniques – capillary microscopy of the hallux nailfold, transcutaneous oximetry of the forefoot, and laser Doppler fluxmetry of the great toe – in a group of 20 patients with hypertension and intermittent claudication or ischemic rest pain, was not affected by the addition of ß-blocking agents.[16] Larger studies[17,18] also suggest that ß-blockers do not reduce peripheral perfusion or adversely affect walking capacity in patients with intermittent claudication and are, in fact, well tolerated in these individuals.

Radack and Deck conducted a meta-analysis of available randomized controlled trials to determine whether or not ß-blockers worsen intermittent claudication. The primary focus of this analysis was the effect of ß-blockers on exercise duration, measured as walking capacity or endurance time. Of the 11 eligible studies, six included individual controlled treatment comparisons that provided data for an analysis of pain-free exercise capacity; no effect size was statistically significant. The pooled effect size for pain-free walking distance was -0.24 (95% CI -0.62 to 0.14), indicating no significant impairment of walking capacity compared with placebo.[18] Only one of the 11 studies reported that ß-blockers may be associated with worsening of intermittent claudication. These results strongly suggest that ß-blockers do not adversely affect walking capacity or symptoms of intermittent claudication in patients with mild-to-moderate PAD.[18] In the absence of other contraindications, ß-blockers should be used in such patients.

Given the adverse prognostic implications of PAD following myocardial infarction, coupled with the known survival benefits of ß-blocker therapy, individuals with PAD might be expected to benefit even more from this form of therapy. Narins et al[14] demonstrated that in postinfarction patients with intermittent claudication, those treated with ß-blocker therapy actually experienced a threefold reduction in cumulative cardiac mortality, compared with patients not treated with ß-blockers (Fig. 6.1). Mukherjee et al demonstrated that, when administered together, the combination of antiplatelet therapy, angiotension-converting enzyme (ACE) inhibitors, ß-blockers, and

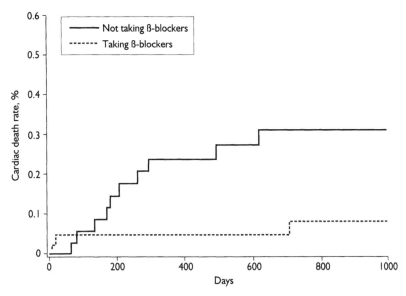

Figure 6.1 *Cumulative probability of cardiac death in postinfarction patients with peripheral arterial disease, taking (n = 43) and not taking (n = 35) β-blockers (p = 0.01, log-rank test). Adapted from Narins et al.*[14]

statins appear to have incremental and maybe even synergistic benefits on cardiovascular morbidity and mortality in patients with PAD as compared to when these agents are administered individually.[19]

More than 44 million non-cardiac surgical procedures are performed in the United States each year,[20] and up to 30% of patients undergoing these procedures either have or are at risk for coronary heart disease, many with evidence of PAD.[21] Patients with PAD have a high incidence of coexisting coronary artery disease.[2] While the rate of perioperative myocardial infarction in patients who do not have coronary disease is estimated to be as low as 0.1–0.7%,[22] the rate of perioperative myocardial infarction in patients with PAD referred for vascular surgery varies between 1 and 37%.[23–25] Studies of acute coronary events in the perioperative period after non-cardiac surgery have suggested that the pathophysiology in at least 50% of patients is due to the disruption of a coronary artery plaque followed by coronary artery thrombosis on this unstable plaque.[26] Recent studies have suggested that aggressive perioperative medical therapy may lower risk in patients who have known coronary disease at the time of major non-cardiac surgery. In several studies the preoperative administration of ß-blockers was associated with a reduction in mortality and cardiovascular complications during and up to 2 years after surgery.[27,28] It is felt that ß-blocker therapy in these patients constitutes the cornerstone of medical therapy.

It appears that the balance of evidence suggests that patients with PAD are a group of patients for whom the use of β-receptor antagonists may impart significant benefit without worsening symptoms of claudication. In the absence of any other absolute contraindications, these drugs should definitely be used when there is concomitant evidence of myocardial ischemia or damage, in the perioperative period of non-cardiac surgery, be considered for the treatment of hypertension in patients with PAD according to established clinical guidelines, and should at least be considered for all other patients with PAD.

Key points

- Beta-blockers do not adversely affect walking capacity or symptoms of intermittent claudication in patients with peripheral arterial disease.
- Beta-blockers significantly reduce cardiovascular morbidity and mortality in patients with peripheral arterial disease.
- Beta-blockers should ideally be administered to all patients perioperatively prior to vascular surgery to reduce cardiovascular morbidity and mortality.

References

1. Frishman WH, Lazar EJ, Gorodokin G. Pharmacokinetic optimisation of therapy with beta-adrenergic blocking agents. Clin Pharmacokinet 1991;20:311–18.

2. Ness J, Aronow WS. Prevalence of coexistence of coronary artery disease, ischemic stroke, and peripheral arterial disease in older persons, mean age 80 years, in an academic hospital-based geriatrics practice. J Am Geriatr Soc 1999;47:1255–6.

3. Weitz JI, Byrne J, Clagett GP, et al. Diagnosis and treatment of chronic arterial insufficiency of the lower extremities: a critical review. Circulation 1996;94:3026–49.

4. Bowlin SJ, Medalie JH, Flocke SA, et al. Intermittent claudication in 8343 men and 21-year specific mortality follow-up. Ann Epidemiol 1997;7:180–7.

5. Muluk SC, Muluk VS, Kelley ME, et al. Outcome events in patients with claudication: a 15-year study in 2777 patients. J Vasc Surg 2001;33:251–7; discussion 257–8.

6. Vogt MT, Cauley JA, Newman AB, Kuller LH, Hulley SB. Decreased ankle/arm blood pressure index and mortality in elderly women. JAMA 1993;270:465–9.

7. Criqui MH, Langer RD, Fronek A, et al. Mortality over a period of 10 years in patients with peripheral arterial disease. N Engl J Med 1992;326:381–6.

8. Hjalmarson A, Elmfeldt D, Herlitz J, et al. Effect on mortality of metoprolol in acute myocardial infarction. A double-blind randomised trial. Lancet 1981;2:823–7.

9. Pedersen TR. Six-year follow-up of the Norwegian Multicenter Study on Timolol after Acute Myocardial Infarction. N Engl J Med 1985;313:1055–8.

10. Gottlieb SS, McCarter RJ, Vogel RA. Effect of beta-blockade on mortality among high-risk and low-risk patients after myocardial infarction. N Engl J Med 1998;339:489–97.

11. Ellerbeck EF, Jencks SF, Radford MJ, et al. Quality of care for Medicare patients with acute myocardial infarction. A four-state pilot study from the Cooperative Cardiovascular Project. JAMA 1995;273:1509–14.

12. Brand DA, Newcomer LN, Freiburger A, Tian H. Cardiologists' practices compared with practice guidelines: use of beta-blockade after acute myocardial infarction. J Am Coll Cardiol 1995;26:1432–6.

13. Viskin S, Kitzis I, Lev E, et al. Treatment with beta-adrenergic blocking agents after myocardial infarction: from randomized trials to clinical practice. J Am Coll Cardiol 1995;25:1327–32.

14. Narins CR, Zareba W, Moss AJ, et al. Relationship between intermittent claudication, inflammation, thrombosis, and recurrent cardiac events among survivors of myocardial infarction. Arch Intern Med 2004;164:440–6.

15. Smith RS, Warren DJ. Effect of beta-blocking drugs on peripheral blood flow in intermittent claudication. J Cardiovasc Pharmacol 1982;4:2–4.

16. Ubbink DT, Verhaar EE, Lie HK, Legemate DA. Effect of beta-blockers on peripheral skin microcirculation in hypertension and peripheral vascular disease. J Vasc Surg 2003;38:535–40.

17. Hiatt WR, Stoll S, Nies AS. Effect of beta-adrenergic blockers on the peripheral circulation in patients with peripheral vascular disease. Circulation 1985;72:1226–31.

18. Radack K, Deck C. Beta-adrenergic blocker therapy does not worsen intermittent claudication in subjects with peripheral arterial disease. A meta-analysis of randomized controlled trials. Arch Intern Med 1991;151:1769–76.

19. Mukherjee D, Lingam P, Chetcuti S, et al. Missed opportunities to treat atherosclerosis in patients undergoing peripheral vascular interventions: insights from the University of Michigan Peripheral Vascular Disease Quality Improvement Initiative (PVD-QI2). Circulation 2002;106:1909–12.

20. Owings MF, Kozak LJ. Ambulatory and inpatient procedures in the United States, 1996. Vital Health Stat 13 1998:1–119.

21. Mangano DT, Goldman L. Preoperative assessment of patients with known or suspected coronary disease. N Engl J Med 1995;333:1750–6.

22. Mangano DT. The cardiac patient and noncardiac surgery: the real challenge. J Cardiothorac Anesth 1987;1:5–6.

23. Boucher CA, Brewster DC, Darling RC, et al. Determination of cardiac risk by dipyridamole-thallium imaging before peripheral vascular surgery. N Engl J Med 1985;312:389–94.

24. Leppo J, Plaja J, Gionet M, et al. Noninvasive evaluation of cardiac risk before elective vascular surgery. J Am Coll Cardiol 1987;9:269–76.

25. Eagle KA, Coley CM, Newell JB, et al. Combining clinical and thallium data optimizes preoperative assessment of cardiac risk before major vascular surgery. Ann Intern Med 1989;110:859–66.

26. Dawood MM, Gutpa DK, Southern J, et al. Pathology of fatal perioperative myocardial infarction: implications regarding pathophysiology and prevention. Int J Cardiol 1996;57:37–44.

27. Mangano DT, Layug EL, Wallace A, Tateo I. Effect of atenolol on mortality and cardiovascular morbidity after noncardiac surgery. Multicenter Study of Perioperative Ischemia Research Group. N Engl J Med 1996;335:1713–20.

28. Poldermans D, Boersma E, Bax JJ, et al. The effect of bisoprolol on perioperative mortality and myocardial infarction in high-risk patients undergoing vascular surgery. Dutch Echocardiographic Cardiac Risk Evaluation Applying Stress Echocardiography Study Group. N Engl J Med 1999;341:1789–94.

7. FIBRINOLYTIC THERAPY IN PERIPHERAL ARTERIAL DISEASE

David S Lee and Deepak L Bhatt

Acute arterial occlusion

Acute lower extremity arterial occlusion presents with the 5 P's: pain, pallor, pulselessness, paresthesias, and paralysis. The incidence of acute arterial ischemia is approximately 14 per 100 000.[1] Acute arterial occlusion is associated with significant morbidity and mortality, including death, limb loss, and extended hospitalizations. Left untreated or treated only by conservative means, the lack of perfusion can result in tissue infarction and necrosis, acidemia, hyperkalemia, myoglobinuria, renal failure, and death. If the ischemic territory does not have perfusion restored quickly enough, amputation may be necessary to save the patient's life.[2] Factors correlating with increased amputation rates in surgical series have included advanced age, concomitant coronary artery disease, extent of peripheral vascular disease, delay in institution of therapy greater than 12 hours, and a greater degree of ischemia at presentation.

Acute peripheral arterial occlusion has traditionally been treated with surgical revascularization. The goal of therapy is to restore perfusion either by restoration of vascular patency using thromboembolectomy or by revascularization using bypass grafting. While this approach has reduced amputation rates and resulted in improved limb salvage, surgical revascularization in this urgent or emergent setting is associated with significant perioperative mortality. This is not primarily because of the ischemia itself, but because of the fragility of this patient cohort and their comorbidities. The lack of tolerance of hemodynamic shifts, general anesthesia, prothrombotic state, and other stresses result in increased cardiovascular and pulmonary complications. In this emergent setting, patients cannot be medically stabilized with anything more than perioperative beta blockade. Improvements in perioperative and postoperative care and surgical techniques have helped but the risks of surgery remain high. Blaisdell et al analyzed the results of 35 case series of patients presenting with acute limb ischemia treated with surgical revascularization and found mortality rates of more than 25%.[3] More recent series still reported mortality rates up to 15–18% with surgical revascularization.[1,4,5] Therefore, fibrinolysis has been pursued as a possible treatment option, so that these patients could be treated with a less-morbid or less-invasive approach or at least stabilized so that elective revascularization could be performed rather than urgent or emergent surgery.

Fibrinolytic therapy

Intra-arterial catheter-directed fibrinolysis restores vessel patency and flow through the dissolution of thrombus or embolus. Intra-arterial fibrinolysis, however, requires an invasive procedure with potential vascular access complications and bleeding complications, the most feared being intracranial hemorrhage. Moreover, the therapy takes hours to restore some arterial flow and potentially greater than 24 hours to achieve full dissolution of thrombus. In the setting of acute limb-threatening ischemia, especially if the ischemia is progressing, the time needed to achieve restoration of flow may be too long and may be associated with tissue infarction and limb loss. In addition, there may still be underlying arterial disease requiring revascularization, although this can usually be achieved either by endovascular means or through simple open surgical procedures: these procedures, if necessary, can be done electively rather than urgently or emergently. Given these limitations, it is clear that only a subset of patients with acute arterial occlusions will benefit from fibrinolysis as opposed to surgical revascularization. The controversy and debate has been deciding which patients will benefit from this therapy. Unfortunately, the studies of fibrinolytic therapy have been somewhat confusing, with conflicting results primarily due to differences in trial design, duration of ischemia, severity of the ischemia, etiology and location of occlusion, and severity of patient comorbidities.

Route of delivery
Systemic
Attempts to infuse fibrinolytic agents intravenously for successful restoration of antegrade flow similar to the use of fibrinolytic agents in acute myocardial infarction have been attempted in the past. Unlike the setting of acute myocardial infarction, however, intravenously administered systemic fibrinolytic therapy has not been successful in the treatment of acute limb ischemia. The large clot burden associated with acute limb ischemia may be less amenable to this type of therapy.

In the early 1970s, uncontrolled clinical studies evaluating approximately 1800 patients treated with fibrinolytic therapy showed at least partial lysis occurring in 40% of patients, with major bleeding complications in approximately 33% of patients. Usually, patients that presented within 72 hours of symptom onset tended to have better success. Overall, intravenous administration of fibrinolysis in this setting has been associated with lower patency rates and higher complication rates compared with intra-arterial fibrinolysis.[6] A more recent study that compared intra-arterial recombinant tissue plasminogen activator (rt-PA) with streptokinase and intravenous rt-PA found that acute patency rates and limb salvage rates were higher in the intra-arterial rt-PA arm and were associated with lower rates of hemorrhage.[7]

Catheter directed intra-arterial fibrinolysis

For fibrinolysis to be effective, the drug must have exposure to the fibrin within the thrombus. In-vitro studies suggest that fibrinolytic agents penetrate organized thrombus very slowly, which probably explains why intravenous administration has had relatively low success rates in achieving reperfusion. Catheter placement within the thrombus, however, with administration of the fibrinolytic agent into the substance of the thrombus, significantly increases the surface area and contact area of the agent to the thrombus while keeping the dose lower, thereby decreasing the risk of bleeding complications. In 1974, Dotter et al first reported the use of streptokinase given intra-arterially at the site of occlusion with successful lysis of the thrombus.[8] Subsequently, several series have suggested that intra-arterial fibrinolysis was associated with higher successful reperfusion rates (50–85%) and lower complication rates. This approach also defined the vascular anatomy, although several visits to the catheterization laboratory were necessary with exposure to contrast and attendant bleeding risks.

Etiology of arterial occlusion

The type or etiology of acute arterial occlusion may be important in determining the success of fibrinolytic therapy. The most common etiologies of acute lower extremity arterial insufficiency or ischemia are arterial thrombosis, arterial embolus, and trauma. Trauma usually causes acute ischemia from vascular damage and occlusion secondary to disruption or laceration. External compression may also lead to vascular obstruction. Iatrogenic vascular trauma and occlusion may occur during arterial catheterization, usually secondary to a flow-limiting dissection. In this setting, surgical repair of the affected vessel is often necessary, although, in some cases, percutaneous techniques may obviate the need for surgery. Fibrinolytic therapy, however, has little utility in treating occlusion secondary to trauma.

Embolic occlusions

Emboli are a common cause of acute lower extremity ischemia, although less frequent than in the past. In approximately 80–85% of cases, the emboli are cardiac in origin,[9] the most common etiologies being secondary to left atrial thrombus from atrial fibrillation or left ventricular thrombus after myocardial infarction.[10] The left atrial appendage is the most common location for thrombus formation in the left atrium, usually as a result of stasis and stagnant blood flow. Acute myocardial infarction can be associated with ventricular thrombus, especially in anterior infarctions. Over time after a myocardial infarction, a ventricular aneurysm can form and lead to thrombus formation. Paradoxical embolism from a patent foramen ovale (PFO) or an atrial septal defect (ASD) can also occur, but is much rarer. Because these emboli are usually organized and may be irregularly shaped, they usually cause incomplete occlusion and ischemia rather than tissue infarction. Also, the underlying arterial bed is often not diseased, as in thrombotic occlusions, with little pre-existing collateral circulation. Therefore, in settings where emboli do cause complete occlusion of the artery, profound acute ischemia leading to tissue loss and infarction may occur and demand immediate intervention.

Arterial emboli from sources other than the heart occur in no more than 20% of cases. The most common are aortic and popliteal artery aneurysms. Emboli from atherosclerotic lesions are rarer. Emboli to the lower extremities are more common than the upper extremities. In one large retrospective series, emboli went to the lower extremity in 63% of cases and to the upper extremity in 20%.[10] The emboli lodge or stop usually at bifurcations or less commonly in areas of atherosclerotic disease with underlying stenosis. The common femoral artery, the common iliac artery, and the popliteal artery, usually at their respective bifurcations, are the most common locations for an acute embolic occlusion.

Patients with embolic phenomenon as the cause of lower extremity ischemia usually have coexisting medical problems, particularly cardiac, including recent myocardial infarction. They may be at higher risk for cardiovascular complications after urgent/emergent vascular surgery. Not surprisingly, in a series of patients presenting with acute lower extremity ischemia either from arterial thrombosis or acute embolism, patients with acute embolism had significantly higher mortality rates.[11] Amputation rates were higher in the patients presenting with arterial thrombosis, however.[12]

Huettl and Soulen reported a retrospective case series of acute arterial occlusions thought secondary to embolization using the Society of Cardiovascular and Interventional Radiology Transluminal Angioplasty and Revascularization (STAT) Registry. There were 45 patients out of 306 total patients in the Registry thought to have embolic occlusions. Only 27% of patients in this series had limb-threatening ischemia. The mean duration of symptoms was 8.6 days. The mean occlusion length was 17 cm. Concomitant coronary artery disease was present in 53% of patients, 40% had prior myocardial infarction, and 50% had atrial fibrillation. Initial technical success was achieved in 69% of patients. A total of 9% of patients died during the follow-up period and 2% required amputation at 30 days. Patency at 1 year in vessels initially treated successfully was 79%. In the University of Rochester trial, short-term event-free survival was similar between acute occlusions caused by embolic or thrombotic occlusions. At 1 year, however, patients with embolic occlusions derived greater benefit when treated with fibrinolysis and overall had higher arterial patency rates, regardless of treatment.[13] Overall, clinical success rates for fibrinolysis for the treatment of arterial embolism causing acute ischemia was approximately 76% ± 15%. This compared favorably to the 81% clinical success rates reported for fibrinolytic treatment for thrombotic occlusions. While these studies are not directly comparable, given different patient populations, presentations, treatment algorithms, etc., the findings suggest that even potentially chronic thrombi which may be organized and more resistant to fibrinolysis may still be amenable to this therapy.

Thrombotic occlusions

Thrombotic occlusions usually occur in the presence of significant underlying atherosclerotic disease. The diseased segments typically are long, but also usually have pre-existing collateral circulation that prevents irreversible limb-threatening ischemia and infarction. In some instances, the collateral blood supply may be so well developed that occlusions may be silent or associated with minimal symptoms. Tissue infarction, gangrene, and rest pain are unusual except in the setting of distal embolization. However, the extent of disease usually means that these patients are more likely to suffer limb loss.[1]

Bypass graft occlusions

The type of vessel in which the occlusion occurs also plays a role in determining the effectiveness of fibrinolytic therapy. Bypass graft occlusions are thought to be more responsive initially to fibrinolytic therapy. Galland et al retrospectively evaluated fibrinolytic therapy in 75 patients with bypass graft occlusions. Overall, graft patency at 1 year after treatment was only 33%. If the lysis was complete with distal vessel runoff, the patency was 39% vs only 17% if the lysis was incomplete.[14] Nehler et al conducted another retrospective analysis in 104 patients with 109 lower extremity bypass occlusions presenting within 14 days of onset of symptoms. Fibrinolytic therapy was successful in restoring patency in 77% of patients. The patency rate at 1 year was 32%, with a limb salvage rate of 73% at 1 year. At 5 years, the patency rate was 19%, while the limb salvage rate was 55%.[15] Overall, initial treatment success is relatively high, but long-term graft patency remains low with patients often requiring further surgical revascularization. However, one meta-analysis evaluating fibrinolytic therapy vs surgery for acute arterial ischemia found that two subgroups that would benefit from fibrinolytic therapy were occlusions of no more than 14 days and occluded bypass grafts.[16]

Severity of ischemia

Patients treated with fibrinolytic therapy must be able to tolerate passage of several hours to achieve reperfusion. If symptoms and critical ischemia are progressing or if the patient has irreversible ischemia (Class III), then immediate surgery is indicated and fibrinolytic therapy should be withheld. The majority of studies evaluating fibrinolytic therapy have enrolled patients presenting with Class I and II ischemia. The severity of presentation and the urgency of therapy will alter the relative risks and benefits of fibrinolytic therapy.

Comparisons between fibrinolytic agents

Physiological fibrinolysis requires cleavage of cross-linked fibrin by active plasmin. Plasminogen is converted to plasmin by endogenous plasminogen activators. Current available thrombolytic, or more accurately, fibrinolytic agents work by activating plasminogen and increasing the activity of the endogenous fibrinolytic system.

Streptokinase is an exogenous plasminogen activator produced by beta-hemolytic Group C streptococci. Streptokinase has proven efficacy in the treatment of ST-segment myocardial infarction; however, it may be less effective than other fibrinolytic agents for acute limb ischemia. Streptokinase is the least expensive fibrinolytic agent but has significant antigenicity from either previous administration of streptokinase or recent streptococcal infection. Antibodies to streptokinase usually result in clearance of and reduced activity of the exogenously administered streptokinase and may also result in allergic reactions.

Urokinase was initially made from human urine. Urokinase is now produced through human tissue culture cells. Although recombinant urokinase was never approved by the Food and Drug Administration (FDA) for use as a fibrinolytic agent in the peripheral circulation, it was widely used until being withdrawn from the market several years ago due to manufacturing issues.[17] Recombinant urokinase is now available again.

Recombinant tissue plasminogen activator (rt-PA) has been evaluated extensively for the treatment of acute myocardial infarction. rt-PA and urokinase have been the most utilized fibrinolytic agents in the treatment of peripheral arterial occlusions. Overall, studies have suggested that both urokinase and rt-PA achieve higher patency rates than streptokinase.[7,18–20] One small randomized trial comparing rt-PA with urokinase found a slight but statistically significant improvement in the recanalization rate with rt-PA for infrainguinal segments.[21]

Reteplase has also been used in this setting but much less commonly than urokinase or rt-PA. The recommended dosages for the commonly used fibrinolytic drugs are listed in Box 7.1. Absolute and relative contraindications to fibrinolytic therapy relate primarily to underlying bleeding risk and are listed in Box 7.2.

Laboratory monitoring after fibrinolysis

Patients are monitored clinically and with laboratory evaluations, including hemoglobin and hematocrit, platelet count, activated partial thromboplastin time, and fibrinogen levels, usually every 6 hours or by clinical changes. Fibrinogen levels have been associated with bleeding complications in some studies but have not been corroborated in larger clinical trials.

Box 7.1 Dosages of commonly used fibrinolytic drugs for peripheral arterial occlusion

Streptokinase (SK)
- Stepwise infusion: SK 1000–3000 IU every 2, 3, 5, 15 min until lysis is complete
- Continuous infusion: SK 5000 – 10 000 IU/h (rarely with initial loading dose of 20 000 or 40 000 IU over 20 min)

Urokinase (UK)
- Stepwise infusion: UK 3000–4000 IU every 3–5 min for stepwise infusion until lysis is complete
- Continuous infusion: 4000 IU/min or up to 100 000 IU/h (occasionally with variable loading dose) until initial recanalization, then 1000–2000 IU/min until complete lysis, all given intra-arterially

Alteplase
- Standard regimen: 0.05–0.1 mg/kg/h intra-arterially or 0.25– 2.5 mg/h
- High-dose regimen: 3 doses of 5.0 mg over 30 min; then 3.5 mg/h for up to 4 h

Reteplase
- 0.25 –1.0 U/h by intra-arterial infusion

Combination therapy
- Reteplase (0.5 U/h) in combination with intravenous administration of abciximab (0.25 mg/kg bolus followed by 0.125 µg/kg/min infusion) for 12 h
- Urokinase initial bolus of 25 000 IU/10 cm of thrombus and continued as an infusion of 4000 IU/min for the first 2 h and 2000 IU/min for 2 more hours if necessary with intravenous administration of abciximab (0.25 mg/kg bolus followed by 0.125 µg/kg/min infusion) for 12 h
- Tenecteplase (5 mg bolus and 0.25 mg/h infusion) and eptifibatide (180 µg/kg bolus and 1 µg/kg/min infusion)

Box 7.2 Contraindications to fibrinolytic therapy

Absolute
1. Established cerebrovascular event (including TIAs within last 2 months)
2. Active bleeding diathesis
3. Recent gastrointestinal bleeding (<10 days)
4. Neurosurgery (intracranial, spinal) within last 3 months
5. Intracranial trauma within last 3 months

Relative major
1. Cardiopulmonary resuscitation within last 10 days
2. Major nonvascular surgery or trauma within last 10 days
3. Uncontrolled hypertension: >180 mmHg systolic or >110 mmHg diastolic
4. Puncture of noncompressible vessel
5. Intracranial tumor
6. Recent eye surgery

Minor
1. Hepatic failure, particularly patients with coagulopathy
2. Bacterial endocarditis
3. Pregnancy
4. Diabetic hemorrhagic retinopathy

Source: from the Working Party on Thrombolysis in the Management of Limb Ischemia Consensus Document.[38]

Randomized trials of fibrinolysis

In the 1980s several retrospective studies were published of patients treated intra-arterially with several fibrinolytic agents, primarily streptokinase, urokinase, and tissue plasminogen activator. The rates of successful recanalization were high. It was not until the 1990s, however, that randomized, clinical trials were conducted to compare surgical revascularization with intra-arterial fibrinolysis.

University of Rochester trial
Ouriel et al conducted the first randomized controlled trial. Intra-arterial fibrinolytic therapy was compared to surgical revascularization as the initial treatment for acute peripheral arterial ischemia. Notably, any underlying lesions discovered angiographically after fibrinolysis underwent definitive

correction. Patients enrolled had to have acute ischemia of less than 7 days' duration. The mean duration of ischemia was less than 24 hours. Patients with embolic or thrombotic occlusions were both included, as were patients with both native arterial and bypass graft occlusions. Importantly, the patients had to have limb-threatening ischemia (Class II). Patients thought to have an embolic etiology were first evaluated by echocardiography to ensure that intracardiac thrombus was not visualized. Patients with intramural thrombus seen on echocardiography were excluded from the study. Patients with either rapidly progressive ischemia requiring emergent treatment or patients with irreversible ischemia (Class III) were not randomized. A total of 114 patients were randomized, 57 into each arm.

Aspirin 325 mg was given orally to all patients after enrollment. Patients in the fibrinolytic therapy arm underwent initial diagnostic angiography, then placement of an infusion catheter directly into the thrombus if technically feasible. Urokinase (Abbokinase, Abbott Laboratories, North Chicago, IL) was infused at a rate of 4000 IU/min for 2 hours, then 2000 IU/min for 2 hours, then 1000 IU/min, up to a maximum of 48 hours. Systemic heparin was not administered during fibrinolytic therapy. Diagnostic angiography was performed at 4, 12, 24, and 48 hours after initiation of therapy.

The primary end points of the study were survival and limb salvage. Event-free survival was defined as amputation-free survival during follow-up. Fibrinolysis of the thrombus was defined to be successful if there was >80% dissolution of thrombus along the entire length of the bypass graft or native artery. Embolism was thought to be the etiology of the acute occlusion in 21% of patients. Of the thrombotic occlusions, 70% involved bypass grafts and 30% involved native arteries. Technical success was achieved in 96% of patients, with arteriographically successful fibrinolysis achieved in 70%. Time to reperfusion was 7.6 ± 0.9 hours with any restoration of flow and a mean duration of 35.6 ± 2.1 hours. A total of 15/17 patients with unsuccessful fibrinolytic therapy underwent operative revascularization and 2/17 patients underwent primary amputation. In hospital cardiopulmonary complications were higher in the surgical revascularization arm (49% vs 16%, $p = 0.001$), with a higher periprocedural myocardial infarction rate (16% vs 5%, $p = 0.02$). One patient had an intracranial hemorrhage that resulted in death. Distal embolization after fibrinolytic therapy occurred in 9% of patients, but in all instances, treatment by repositioning the catheter and continuing fibrinolytic therapy resulted in complete dissolution of the embolus. The duration of hospitalization was not different between the two groups, with a median length of stay equal to 11 days. Cumulative amputation-free survival was significantly better in the fibrinolytic group (84% vs 58%, $p = 0.01$) at 1 year. Notably, the cumulative risk of amputation was similar between the two groups, at 18%. Multivariate analysis revealed only one variable, besides treatment allocation that was predictive of death. Patients with Goldman classes 3 and 4 in their perioperative risk assessment had a higher mortality rate (relative risk (RR) 1.65, 95% CI 1.15–2.32).[13]

Fibrinolytic therapy in this cohort of patients was associated with improved survival. It is likely that the significant comorbidities and pre-existing cardiac disease were the major determinants of increased perioperative mortality in the surgery group. The acuity of presentation (within 24 hours on average) probably contributed to the success of fibrinolytic therapy.

TOPAS trial

The Thrombolysis or Peripheral Arterial Surgery (TOPAS) trial was a multicenter, randomized, clinical trial that evaluated fibrinolysis using recombinant urokinase (rUK) vs surgical revascularization for the initial treatment of patients with acute limb-threatening lower extremity arterial occlusion. Patients in the TOPAS trial had to have Class II (reversible limb-threatening) ischemia – as defined by the Society for Vascular Surgery/International Society for Cardiovascular Surgery. Symptoms not only had to be severe but also had to be of less than 14 days in duration. Patients with both thrombotic and embolic etiologies were enrolled, as were patients with both native artery and bypass graft occlusions. Initially, a phase I dose-ranging trial was conducted to determine the optimal dose of urokinase to achieve dissolution of thrombus and restoration of vessel patency. In the TOPAS phase I dose-ranging trial, in 213 patients with acute lower extremity ischemia, a regimen of 4000 IU/min for 4 hours, followed by 2000 IU/min thereafter for up to an additional 44 hours, resulted in thrombus dissolution in 71% of patients, with the lowest complication rate of the three infusion regimens tested.[22]

In the TOPAS trial phase II, the primary end point of the trial was amputation-free survival at 6 months. The average age was 64.7 years old. The fibrinolytic therapy group was more likely to be male, have hepatic or renal insufficiency, and was more likely to present with rest pain at presentation. Embolism was the etiology in only 15%. The average length of occlusion was approximately 32 cm (15–25 cm in native arterial occlusions and 38–47 cm in graft occlusions). A total of 42% of patients had concomitant coronary artery disease. The mean duration of symptoms was slightly greater than 4 days. Technical success was achieved in 85% of patients. The mean duration of urokinase infusion was 24.4 ± 0.86 hours. Open surgical procedures were avoided in 46% of patients in the urokinase group.

In the phase II study, concomitant unfractionated heparin was also infused with recombinant urokinase, with a target activated partial thromboplastin time (aPTT) of 1.5–2 times control value. The first 62 patients treated with this regimen had a 4.8% intracranial hemorrhage rate; therefore, the data safety monitoring committee modified the regimen so that therapeutic doses of intravenous heparin as well as initial aspirin therapy were both contraindicated. These findings again demonstrate the relatively low therapeutic index of fibrinolytic therapy, especially in the setting of systemic anticoagulation.[23]

Restoration of some flow was seen in 79.7% of patients, while complete thrombus dissolution was observed in 67.9%. Amputation-free survival rates were 71.8% in the fibrinolytic group vs 74.8% in the surgery group ($p = 0.43$). At 1 year, it was 65.0% vs 69.9% respectively ($p = 0.23$). At hospital discharge the mortality rate for fibrinolytic therapy was 8.8% vs 5.9% for surgical revascularization ($p = 0.19$). The length of stay (LOS) was similar between groups, with a median LOS of 10 days in each treatment group. The risk of major bleeding was 12.5% in the fibrinolytic arm vs 5.5% in the surgical arm ($p = 0.005$). Four patients (1.6%) had intracranial hemorrhage. In this study, fibrinolysis was associated with fewer open surgical procedures, allowing approximately 50% of patients to avoid surgery entirely, without an increase in mortality or amputation rates. The duration of hospitalization remained the same.[23]

This trial showed discordant results with the Rochester study, but the findings are probably representative of differences in patient characteristics and presentation. The severity of limb ischemia was greater in the Rochester trial than in the TOPAS trial and the duration of symptoms was shorter. Moreover, the Rochester study patients tended to be older, with greater incidence of coronary artery disease. Overall, the patients in the Rochester trial were probably at higher perioperative risk than patients in the TOPAS trial.

STILE trial

The Surgery versus Thrombolysis for Ischemia of the Lower Extremity (STILE) trial was a prospective randomized clinical trial comparing catheter-directed fibrinolysis to surgical revascularization in patients presenting with lower extremity arterial ischemia of less than 6 months' duration. The etiology had to be non-embolic, with occlusions in either native arteries or bypass grafts. A total of 393 patients were enrolled before the trial was stopped because a primary end point had been met during interim analysis. A significant higher rate of recurrent or ongoing ischemia was seen in the fibrinolytic-treated group ($p <0.001$). A post hoc analysis stratified patients by duration of ischemia (greater than 14 days vs less than or equal to 14 days). Patients with less than or equal to 14 days of ischemia had a trend for lower amputation rates ($p = 0.052$) with fibrinolytic therapy, whereas patients with greater than 14 days of ischemia had less ongoing or recurrent ischemia with surgical treatment ($p <0.001$) with a trend for lower mortality ($p = 0.1$).[24]

In long-term results reported from this study, 237 patients with native arterial occlusions were treated with either surgery or fibrinolysis with urokinase or tissue plasminogen activator. A total of 150 patients were treated with catheter-directed fibrinolysis (84 patients with rt-PA and 66 patients with rUK) and 87 patients underwent surgical revascularization; 69 patients had iliac artery or common femoral artery occlusion and 168 patients had superficial femoral artery (SFA) or popliteal artery occlusion. The primary end points of the trial were recurrent ischemia, morbidity, amputation, and death rates at 30 days, 6 months, and 1 year. Importantly, patients had to have new or progressive ischemia symptoms starting within the past 6 months. Before they could be enrolled, an angiogram must have demonstrated a non-embolic occlusion. A total of 78% of patients randomized to catheter-directed fibrinolysis had successful placement of the catheter into the occluded artery and infusion of the fibrinolytic agent. Patients' presenting symptoms were rest pain in 35% and ischemic ulceration or tissue necrosis in 31%. Notably, 34% of patients presented with claudication. The mean duration of symptoms was 59 days. Approximately 20% had symptoms of less than 2 weeks in duration. There were no significant differences between the baseline characteristics in the fibrinolytic and surgery groups. Fibrinolytic therapy restored flow and vessel patency in 55% of patients (49% with UK and 59% with rt-PA, no significant difference). The time to achieve lysis, however, was lower in the rt-PA group (8 hours vs 24 hours, p <0.05). A secondary procedure was required in 55% of patients treated with fibrinolysis, 75% being endovascular procedures. Surgical revascularization primarily consisted of bypass grafting (86% of patients).[25]

At 1 year, ongoing and recurrent ischemia (defined as no improvement in perfusion or recurrent thrombosis of successful procedure) was significantly higher in the fibrinolytic group (64% vs 35%, p <0.0001). Furthermore, major amputation was also higher in the fibrinolytic group (10% vs 0%, p = 0.0024), although mortality rates were not significantly different. Severity of limb ischemia and diabetes mellitus, however, were significant factors associated with the success of thrombolytic therapy, especially in the cohort of patients with SFA–popliteal artery occlusions. In these patients, treatment with thrombolysis was associated with improved survival, albeit with increased rates of recurrent ischemia and amputation. The duration of symptoms may be important in the success of fibrinolytic therapy, and the results of STILE would suggest that fibrinolytic therapy may not be as favorable in subacute and chronic lesions (80% of patients in STILE had duration of symptoms between 14 days and 6 months).[25]

Bleeding complications

The Rochester study reported 11% major bleeding and one intracranial hemorrhage. In the TOPAS trial, there was a 12.5% rate of major bleeding, with 1.6% rate of intracranial hemorrhage, and an increased risk if patients received concomitant intravenous unfractionated heparin. The STILE study reported a 5.6% occurrence of major bleeding. Overall, in a summary of 19 prospective series, the risk of stroke was 1.0%, major hemorrhage 5.1%, and minor hemorrhage 14.8%.[26]

Conclusions from the clinical trials of fibrinolytic therapy

These trials show the heterogeneity of patients and presentations that make conclusions about the role of fibrinolysis for lower extremity arterial occlusions difficult. The trials do not show unequivocal evidence that fibrinolysis is associated with lower mortality rates or higher limb salvage rates. The use of intra-arterial fibrinolysis must be thought of as one potential option/therapy in the armamentarium of possible treatments for acute limb ischemia. Currently, the exact role of fibrinolysis is still being defined.

An initial meta-analysis performed in 1996 found that intra-arterial fibrinolysis was associated with improved survival. The mortality at 30 days was 4% for fibrinolysis vs 15% for surgery. Limb salvage rates were 93% and 86%, respectively.[27] However, a more recent meta-analysis of 10 randomized controlled trials of fibrinolysis vs surgery found similar rates of major amputation (relative risk for fibrinolysis vs surgery RR 0.893, 95% CI 0.576–1.383) and mortality (RR 1.24, 95% CI 0.795–1.9). Fibrinolytic therapy was, however, associated with an increased risk of bleeding (RR 2.94, 95% CI 1.1–7.9). Multivariate analysis found that occlusions of no more than 14 days and occluded bypass grafts may benefit from fibrinolysis.[16] Another meta-analysis of five trials with 1283 patients found that rates of limb salvage and mortality were similar between fibrinolysis and surgery at 30 days, 6 months, and 1 year. Fibrinolytic therapy was associated with an elevated stroke risk at 30 days (OR 6.41, 95% CI 1.57–26.22) and a higher rate of major bleeding (OR 2.80, 95% CI 1.70–4.60) but with a lesser degree of intervention required for revascularization (OR 5.37, 95% CI 3.99–7.22). The increased risk of major bleeding, including hemorrhagic stroke, should be balanced against the risk of surgery in any given patient.[28]

Overall, catheter-directed intra-arterial fibrinolytic therapy can be utilized to successfully recanalize and reperfuse arterial occlusions. The success of this technique is higher when patients are treated within 2 weeks of symptom onset, although chronic lesions may respond, but to a lesser extent. In the majority of settings, further endovascular procedures or open surgery will probably be needed to consolidate the results of fibrinolysis and to achieve more durable revascularization. Notably, distal occlusions in small arterial beds may be more successfully treated with fibrinolysis.

Chronic total occlusions

The role of fibrinolytic agents in the treatment of chronic arterial occlusions is controversial. Fibrinolysis may dissolve thrombus and reduce the length of occluded segments. McNamara reported a series of patients with chronic occlusions treated with intra-arterial fibrinolysis, with recanalization in nearly half of the patients.[29] Subsequent endovascular procedures were used.

Future of fibrinolysis

Newer agents

Recombinant prourokinase is being studied as a fibrinolytic agent with improved fibrin specificity. A recent randomized multicenter phase II study evaluated three different doses of recombinant prourokinase compared to a standard regimen of urokinase in the treatment of acute lower extremity peripheral arterial occlusion of less than or equal to 14 days. This study found that the highest dose of prourokinase (8 mg/h for 8 hours then 0.5 mg/h) was associated with increased clot lysis, decreased fibrinogen concentrations, and mildly increased bleeding vs the other treatment groups. Further studies will be necessary to ascertain the potential uses of recombinant prourokinase.[30]

Alfimeprase (Nuvelo, Sunnyvale, CA) is a novel fibrinolytic that is beginning an extensive round of clinical testing. It is a recombinant enzyme that appears to dissolve clots very quickly and may represent a major advance in catheter-directed fibrinolysis. Additionally, alfimeprase is rapidly inactivated by alpha-2 macroglobulin in the blood, and therefore may prove to have much less in the way of systemic bleeding risk, potentially including a much lower risk of intracranial hemorrhage.

Glycoprotein IIb/IIIa inhibitors and combination therapy

Glycoprotein IIb/IIIa inhibitors have been used as successful adjuncts to fibrinolytic therapy for the treatment of ST-elevation myocardial infarction. The use of these agents as combination therapy in the setting of acute lower extremity arterial occlusion is significantly less well studied. A pilot study treated 15 patients with acute and subacute lower extremity arterial occlusions with catheter-directed intra-arterial reteplase infusions with intravenous abciximab for 12 hours. Complete angiographic clot dissolution occurred in 14/15 patients (93%), with a 30-day patency rate of 93%. The mean time to achieve lysis was 17.5 hours. This pilot study suggested that combination therapy is possible, but further trials will be necessary.[31] A small retrospective study also found similar findings with eptifibatide. Combination therapy was associated with similar efficacy and safety with a decrease in the dose of rt-PA required to achieve clot lysis.[32] In the Platelet Receptor Antibodies in Order to Manage Peripheral Artery Thrombosis (PROMPT) study, 70 patients with arterial occlusions of less than 6 weeks' duration were treated with either urokinase or urokinase plus abciximab. Combination therapy achieved faster clot lysis, with a trend towards an increased rate of major bleeding. Amputation-free survival at 3 months was 96% in the combination therapy arm vs 80% in the urokinase alone arm ($p = 0.04$).[33] Economic analysis of this trial revealed that combination therapy accrued lower direct medical costs at 3 months than urokinase alone.[34]

Pulse-spray thrombolysis

Modifications to catheter-directed fibrinolytic therapy were attempted to improve the speed and extent of thrombus dissolution. Pulse-spray delivery of fibrinolytic agents utilized multiple short bursts of the agent into the thrombus to potentially increase channel formation and area of contact. Yusuf et al evaluated pulse-spray thrombolysis using rt-PA in 24 patients presenting with lower extremity ischemia. The mean duration of treatment was 137.5 min, with complete angiographic lysis occurring in 96% of the patients treated. The 30-day mortality was 16.6%, and 75% of patients treated had limb salvage at 30 days.[35] Another small study found the median fibrinolytic infusion time to be 195 min for the pulse-spray arm vs 1390 min for conventional intra-arterial fibrinolysis.[36] Armon et al studied pulse-spray thrombolysis in acute and subacute lower extremity ischemia using rt-PA. Median duration of lysis was 135 min, with complete angiographic lysis seen in 79%. The cumulative limb salvage rate was 79% at 30 months. Major bleeding occurred in 7% and minor bleeding occurred in 24%.[37] It is theoretically possible that this technique may be associated with increased distal embolization of partially lysed thrombus. Overall, this technique shows potential for more rapid clot dissolution and may potentially expand the use of fibrinolytic therapy. Further trials, however, are needed.

Conclusion

Fibrinolytic therapy has significantly evolved over the past four decades. The benefit of fibrinolysis may ultimately be for a select group of patients presenting early with arterial thrombosis as the etiology of their acute limb ischemia that are threatened but not at emergent amputation risk with multiple comorbidities and at elevated surgical risk. Newer adjuvant pharmacological therapies and new endovascular techniques to infuse fibrinolytic therapy may broaden the indications for fibrinolytic therapy in the near future.

> **Key points**
> - Acute lower extremity arterial occlusion presents with the **5 P's**: pain, pallor, pulselessness, paresthesias, and paralysis.
> - Patients who suffer acute arterial thrombi or emboli should be systemically heparinized to prevent proximal and distal thrombotic propagation. Heparin followed by oral anticoagulation should be used to prevent recurrent embolism in patients undergoing thromboembolectomy.
> - Optimal patient outcome depends on the rapidity and completeness with which arterial blood flow to the limb can be re-established
> - Intra-arterial thrombolytic therapy may be considered in patients with acute (less than 14 days) thrombotic or embolic occlusive disease provided that there is a low risk of myonecrosis developing during the time to achieve revascularization by this method.
> - Newer adjuvant pharmacological therapies and endovascular techniques to infuse fibrinolytic therapy may broaden the indications for fibrinolytic therapy in the future.

References

1. Dormandy J, Heeck L, Vig S. Acute limb ischemia. Semin Vasc Surg 1999;12:148–53.

2. Blaisdell FW. The pathophysiology of skeletal muscle ischemia and the reperfusion syndrome: a review. Cardiovasc Surg 2002;10:620–30.

3. Blaisdell FW, Steele M, Allen RE. Management of acute lower extremity arterial ischemia due to embolism and thrombosis. Surgery 1978;84:822–34.

4. Yeager RA, Moneta GL, Taylor LM Jr, et al. Surgical management of severe acute lower extremity ischemia. J Vasc Surg 1992;15:385–91; discussion 392–3.

5. Tawes RL Jr, Harris EJ, Brown WH, et al. Arterial thromboembolism. A 20-year perspective. Arch Surg 1985;120:595–9.

6. Boyles PW, Meyer WH, Graff J, Ashley CC, Ripic RG. Comparative effectiveness of intravenous and intra-arterial fibrinolysin therapy. Am J Cardiol 1960;6:439–46.

7. Berridge DC, Gregson RH, Hopkinson BR, Makin GS. Randomized trial of intra-arterial recombinant tissue plasminogen activator, intravenous recombinant tissue plasminogen activator and intra-arterial streptokinase in peripheral arterial thrombolysis. Br J Surg 1991;78:988–95.

8. Dotter CT, Rosch J, Seaman AJ. Selective clot lysis with low-dose streptokinase. Radiology 1974;111:31–7.

9. Elliott JP, Jr, Hageman JH, Szilagyi E, et al. Arterial embolization: problems of source, multiplicity, recurrence, and delayed treatment. Surgery 1980;88:833–45.

10. Abbott WM, Maloney RD, McCabe CC, Lee CE, Wirthlin LS. Arterial embolism: a 44 year perspective. Am J Surg 1982;143:460–4.

11. Brewster DC. Acute peripheral arterial occlusion. Cardiol Clin 1991;9:497–513.

12. Cambria RP, Abbott WM. Acute arterial thrombosis of the lower extremity. Its natural history contrasted with arterial embolism. Arch Surg 1984;119:784–7.

13. Ouriel K, Shortell CK, DeWeese JA, et al. A comparison of thrombolytic therapy with operative revascularization in the initial treatment of acute peripheral arterial ischemia. J Vasc Surg 1994;19:1021–30.

14. Galland RB, Magee TR, Whitman B, et al. Patency following successful thrombolysis of occluded vascular grafts. Eur J Vasc Endovasc Surg 2001;22:157–60.

15. Nehler MR, Mueller RJ, McLafferty RB, et al. Outcome of catheter-directed thrombolysis for lower extremity arterial bypass occlusion. J Vasc Surg 2003;37:72–8.

16. Palfreyman SJ, Booth A, Michaels JA. A systematic review of intra-arterial thrombolytic therapy for lower-limb ischaemia. Eur J Vasc Endovasc Surg 2000;19:143–57.

17. Ouriel K. Current status of thrombolysis for peripheral arterial occlusive disease. Ann Vasc Surg 2002;16:797–804.

18. van Breda A, Katzen BT, Deutsch AS. Urokinase versus streptokinase in local thrombolysis. Radiology 1987;165:109–11.

19. Meyerovitz MF, Goldhaber SZ, Reagan K, et al. Recombinant tissue-type plasminogen activator versus urokinase in peripheral arterial and graft occlusions: a randomized trial. Radiology 1990;175:75–8.

20. Dawson KJ, Reddy K, Platts AD, Hamilton G. Results of a recently instituted programme of thrombolytic therapy in acute lower limb ischaemia. Br J Surg 1991;78:409–11.

21. Schweizer J, Altmann E, Stosslein F, Florek HJ, Kaulen R. Comparison of tissue plasminogen activator and urokinase in the local infiltration thrombolysis of peripheral arterial occlusions. Eur J Radiol 1996;22:129–32.

22. Ouriel K, Veith FJ, Sasahara AA. Thrombolysis or peripheral arterial surgery: phase I results. TOPAS Investigators. J Vasc Surg 1996;23:64–73; discussion 74–5.

23. Ouriel K, Veith FJ, Sasahara AA. A comparison of recombinant urokinase with vascular surgery as initial treatment for acute arterial occlusion of the legs. Thrombolysis or Peripheral Arterial Surgery (TOPAS) Investigators. N Engl J Med 1998;338:1105–11.

24. Results of a prospective randomized trial evaluating surgery versus thrombolysis for ischemia of the lower extremity. The STILE trial. Ann Surg 1994;220:251–66; discussion 266–8.

25. Weaver FA, Comerota AJ, Youngblood M, et al. Surgical revascularization versus thrombolysis for nonembolic lower extremity native artery occlusions: results of a prospective randomized trial. The STILE Investigators. Surgery versus Thrombolysis for Ischemia of the Lower Extremity. J Vasc Surg 1996;24:513–21; discussion 521–3.

26. Berridge DC, Makin GS, Hopkinson BR. Local low dose intra-arterial thrombolytic therapy: the risk of stroke or major haemorrhage. Br J Surg 1989;76:1230–3.

27. Diffin DC, Kandarpa K. Assessment of peripheral intraarterial thrombolysis versus surgical revascularization in acute lower-limb ischemia: a review of limb-salvage and mortality statistics. J Vasc Interv Radiol 1996;7:57–63.

28. Berridge DC, Kessel D, Robertson I. Surgery versus thrombolysis for acute limb ischaemia: initial management. Cochrane Database Syst Rev 2002:CD002784.

29. McNamara TO. Role of thrombolysis in peripheral arterial occlusion. Am J Med. 1987;83:6–10.

30. Ouriel K, Kandarpa K, Schuerr DM, et al. Prourokinase versus urokinase for recanalization of peripheral occlusions, safety and efficacy: the PURPOSE trial. J Vasc Interv Radiol 1999;10:1083–91.

31. Drescher P, Crain MR, Rilling WS. Initial experience with the combination of reteplase and abciximab for thrombolytic therapy in peripheral arterial occlusive disease: a pilot study. J Vasc Interv Radiol 2002;13:37–43.

32. Yoon HC, Miller FJ, Jr. Using a peptide inhibitor of the glycoprotein IIb/IIIa platelet receptor: initial experience in patients with acute peripheral arterial occlusions. AJR Am J Roentgenol 2002;178:617–22.

33. Duda SH, Tepe G, Luz O, et al. Peripheral artery occlusion: treatment with abciximab plus urokinase versus with urokinase alone – a randomized pilot trial (the PROMPT Study). Platelet Receptor Antibodies in Order to Manage Peripheral Artery Thrombosis. Radiology 2001;221:689–96.

34. Duda SH, Tepe G, Bala M, et al. Economic value of thrombolysis with adjunctive abciximab in patients with subacute peripheral arterial occlusion. Pharmacoeconomics 2002;20:203–13.

35. Yusuf SW, Whitaker SC, Gregson RH, et al. Experience with pulse-spray technique in peripheral thrombolysis. Eur J Vasc Surg 1994;8:270–5.

36. Yusuf SW, Whitaker SC, Gregson RH, et al. Prospective randomised comparative study of pulse spray and conventional local thrombolysis. Eur J Vasc Endovasc Surg 1995;10:136–41.

37. Armon MP, Yusuf SW, Whitaker SC, et al. Results of 100 cases of pulse-spray thrombolysis for acute and subacute leg ischaemia. Br J Surg 1997;84:47–50.

38. Working Party on Thrombolysis in the Management of Limb Ischemia Thrombolysis in the management of lower limb peripheral arterial occlusion – a consensus document. J Vasc Interv Radiol 2003;14:S337–49.

8. ANTITHROMBOTIC THERAPIES

Marco Roffi

Introduction

Antiplatelet and antithrombotic agents (anticoagulants) are mainstays in the treatment of peripheral arterial disease (PAD). Much of the knowledge on antithrombotic therapies is derived from percutaneous coronary intervention and acute coronary syndromes.[1] In patients with chronic disease, the first goal of antiplatelet therapy is the overall reduction of cardiovascular events. To a lesser extent, these agents are helpful in reducing local disease progression and arterial occlusion. The need for long-term oral anticoagulation is limited to a high-risk subset of patients following surgical revascularization of the lower extremities. During percutaneous transluminal angioplasty (PTA), both antiplatelet agents and anticoagulants have a critical role in the prevention of thromboembolic events associated with the procedure. The present chapter will focus on anticoagulants, while antiplatelet and fibrinolytic-based therapies are addressed in Chapter 3 and Chapter 7, respectively.

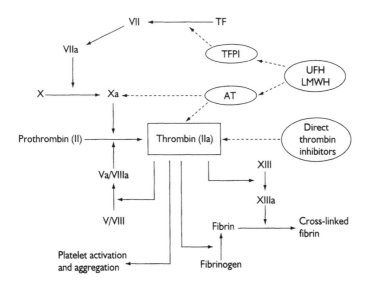

Figure 8.1 *Pathogenesis of clot formation and target sites of anticoagulants.*
AT = antithrombin; LMWH = low-molecular-weight heparin; TF = tissue factor;
TFPI = tissue factor pathway inhibitor; UFH = unfractionated heparin.

Thrombin plays a key role in thrombus formation (Fig. 8.1). Thrombin generation represents the culmination of the coagulation cascade. Among its numerous procoagulant and prothrombotic actions, thrombin converts fibrinogen to fibrin and activates factor XIII to XIIIa, which in turn cross-link fibrin into a stable, insoluble clot. Moreover, thrombin regulates its own production by activating factor V to Va and factor VIII to VIIIa, both of which in turn promote thrombin and clot generation.[2] This positive feedback activation causes a non-linear generation of thrombin. Additionally, this molecule is a potent stimulus for platelet activation, adhesion, and aggregation. Thrombin also stimulates endogenous thrombolysis via release of tissue plasminogen activator (t-PA). When prothrombin is converted to thrombin, it releases prothrombin F_{1+2} fragment. Measures of prothrombin F_{1+2} fragment thus reflect thrombin generation.[3] When thrombin catalyzes the proteolysis of fibrinogen to fibrin, fibrinopeptide A (a short polypeptide remnant) is released and, when measured, is an index of thrombin activity.[3] Finally, thrombin has also vasoactive properties, inducing vasodilation in vessels with intact endothelium and vasoconstriction in vessels with damaged endothelium.[2]

On a molecular level, thrombin is a serine protease with several distinct recognition sites, including the catalytic binding site, an anion-binding exosite, an apolar binding site, and separate sites at which binding to unfractioned heparin (UFH) and fibrin occurs (Fig. 8.2).[4] The catalytic binding site is the active center triggering conversion of fibrinogen to fibrin. Direct thrombin inhibitors such as bivalirudin bind at both the catalytic site and the substrate recognition (anion-binding site) (see Fig. 8.2).

Pharmacological principles of anticoagulation in peripheral arterial disease

Unfractionated heparin

UFH, which is extracted from bovine lung or porcine intestinal mucosa, is a glycosaminoglycan made up of polysaccharide chains, ranging in molecular weight from 3000 to 30 000 Da. Since UFH is a macromolecule, it is not absorbed by the gastrointestinal tract. When injected subcutaneously, the bioavailability of UFH ranges from 10% to 90%, depending on the dose given; therefore intravenous application is preferred. However, with intravenous application, the anticoagulant effect is unpredictable due to poor and markedly variable bioavailability caused by its propensity to bind to plasma proteins, endothelial cells, platelets, and macrophages (Table 8.1).[5] As a consequence, frequent assessment of the level of anticoagulation is necessary. Additional potential disadvantages of UFH include its inability to inactivate clot-bound thrombin, probably owing to a conformational change in thrombin's structure and protection once bound to fibrin (see Fig. 8.2).[6]

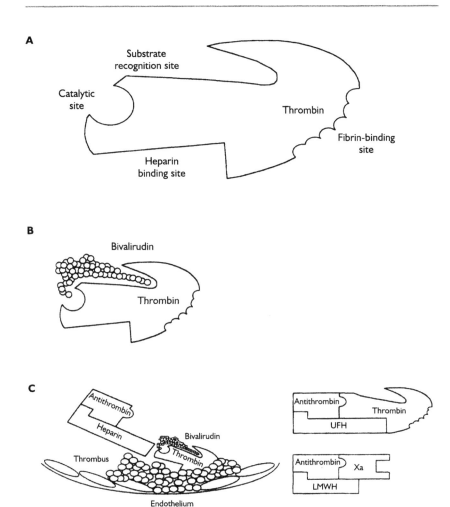

Figure 8.2 (A) Schematic of the thrombin molecule, which is a complex protein containing several specialized receptor sites, including the substrate recognition site (anion binding) and active catalytic site as well as separate sites where binding to fibrin and heparin occur. (B) Direct thrombin inhibitors such as bivalirudin bind the thrombin molecule over an extended region, covering the sites on the molecule that are involved in substrate recognition as well as the catalytic site. (C) Unfractionated heparin (UFH), an indirect thrombin inhibitor, cannot inactivate clot-bound thrombin, probably owing to a conformational change in thrombin's structure and protection once bound to fibrin. Direct thrombin inhibitors (e.g. bivalirudin) are smaller molecules, require no cofactors, and can reach the substrate or catalytic sites of thrombin within the thrombus. Low-molecular-weight heparins (LMWHs) preferentially bind to factor Xa because of their shorter saccharide lengths. (Reproduced with permission from Lauer et al.[39])

103

Table 8.1 Pharmacological properties of anticoagulants

Unfractionated heparin	Low-molecular-weight heparin	Direct thrombin inhibitor
Inhibits thrombin and factor Xa	Mainly inhibits factor Xa	Inhibits thrombin
Does not inactivate clot-bound thrombin	Does not inactivate clot-bound thrombin	Inactivates clot-bound thrombin
Anticoagulation fairly unpredictable	Anticoagulation more predictable	Anticoagulation more predictable
Elimination: reticuloendothelial system	Elimination: renal	Elimination: renal
Monitoring required	Generally, no monitoring is required	Monitoring required
Can be completely neutralized	Can be partially neutralized	Cannot be neutralized

Accordingly, UFH blood concentrations in the therapeutic range, although able to completely inhibit fluid-phase thrombin, only produce 20–40% inhibition of clot-bound thrombin. Similarly, in-vitro studies have shown that a 20-fold higher concentration of UFH is needed to block 70% of activity in the clot-bound enzyme than is required for equivalent inhibition of fluid-phase thrombin.[7] It is unknown whether these mechanisms are of any clinical relevance in the treatment of patients with PAD. However, the usually short duration of UFH therapy (e.g. periprocedurally or as bridging to oral anticoagulation) makes it unlikely that the mentioned limitations have a clinical impact.

The same is true for a serious side effect of UFH, namely heparin-induced thrombocytopenia (HIT). Data from the coronary experience show that after 1–4 days of therapy, approximately 10–20% of patients develop transient mild thrombocytopenia (platelet count rarely below 100 000/μl).[8] Clinically manifest HIT, characterized by medium-to-large vessel thrombotic occlusion, leading to widespread thrombosis and gangrene, is rare but is associated with significant morbidity and mortality. No data are available on the incidence of HIT among patients treated with UFH for PAD.

Low-molecular-weight heparins

Low-molecular-weight heparins (LMWHs) are salts of sulfated glycosaminoglycan with molecular mass distribution ranging between 4300 and 5800 Da. They are obtained by fractionation or depolymerization of UFH. Individual LMWHs differ with respect to bioavailability, anti-factor Xa (anti-Xa) and anti-factor IIa (anti-IIa) activities, anti-Xa:anti-IIa ratio, antithrombotic potency, capacity to release endothelial tissue factor pathway inhibitor (TFPI), and bleeding profile.[9] Patients with renal insufficiency have delayed clearance of LMWH, with no strict correlation to the severity of the kidney disease. Although a dose adjustment in this setting is recommended, there are minimal data to guide therapy.

LMWH shows several advantages compared with UFH (see Table 8.1): the anticoagulation with LMWH is more predictable, no monitoring is required in the absence of major renal dysfunction, there is no dose-dependent clearance, less binding to plasma proteins, and no evidence of platelet stimulation. As a result of these properties, a predictable anticoagulant effect may be achieved at a fixed dose with no need for laboratory resources. Furthermore, with LMWH there is a higher ratio of factor Xa to factor IIa inhibition, indicating that the coagulation cascade is inhibited further upstream with potent inhibition of thrombin generation as well as inhibition of thrombin activity. Regarding safety, thrombocytopenia (HIT) is less frequently encountered than with UFH.[10] Because of its pharmacokinetic properties, the dose–response curve of LMWH tends to be linear. This observation implies that the anticoagulation effect of a given dose should be highly predictable, lessening the need for monitoring. Current recommendations include no routine laboratory monitoring of a weight-adjusted, fixed-dose LMWH regimen. Although it may be mildly prolonged during therapy, the activated partial thromboplastin time (aPTT) and the activated clotting time (ACT) are not helpful in monitoring LMWH. As no comparative studies have been performed, it is unknown whether these theoretical advantages of LMWH over UFH translate into a benefit for patients with PAD (e.g. in the setting of PTA or as a bridging to oral anticoagulation).

Common limitations of UFH and LMWH

One major limiting factor of both UFH and LMWH is their inability to inhibit thrombin that is bound to fibrin. Neither UFH-antithrombin nor LMWH-antithrombin are effective inhibitors of fibrin-bound thrombin because the UFH-binding site on thrombin is masked when the enzyme is bound to fibrin (see Fig. 8.2).[6] In the coronary circulation, it has been postulated that this property may limit the effectiveness of UFH, and possibly of LMWH, particularly when there is a delay from clinical presentation to administration of drug in the setting of acute coronary syndromes. Antithrombin-independent direct thrombin inhibitors such as bivalirudin, which effectively inhibit fibrin-bound as well as free thrombin, may be more effective in this clinical setting.[6] Numerous pharmacological differences have been observed between LMWHs that have the potential to influence efficacy. However, no head-to-head

105

comparison among LMWHs has been performed thus far, neither in the coronary nor in the peripheral vasculature. Therefore, the clinical relevance of such findings remains unknown.

Direct thrombin inhibitors

Lepirudin is the prototype of direct thrombin inhibitors. It binds tightly to thrombin and blocks both its active (catalytic) site and its substrate-binding site, and also establishes close contact over an extended surface of the thrombin molecule, thereby inactivating all known functions of thrombin (see Fig. 8.2).[3] Bivalirudin is synthesized by combining a peptide fragment of lepirudin (hirugen), which is a weak thrombin inhibitor, with a tetrapeptide specific for inhibiting the catalytic site of thrombin. Direct thrombin inhibitors offer several potential advantages over UFH (see Table 8.1). They are specific and potent inhibitors of thrombin, acting independently from antithrombin and other endogenous factors. Unlike UFH, direct thrombin inhibitors are able to inhibit clot-bound thrombin both in vitro and in vivo.[6,11] Direct thrombin inhibitors do not bind to the endothelium or macrophages and produce more stable level of anticoagulation over time. They do not cause HIT nor do they cross-react with the antibodies that cause HIT and therefore have been reported to be useful in patients with HIT who require continued anticoagulation.[12]

A clear disadvantage of these compounds is the lack of a reversal agent. Moreover, direct thrombin inhibitors appear to be a relatively more potent inhibitor of thrombin action but a less effective inhibitor of thrombin generation than UFH.[11] Plasma bivalirudin concentrations correlate well with aPTT levels, and at present aPTT is considered the test of choice for monitoring therapy.[13] Conversely, no strong correlation was found between bivalirudin levels and ACT.[14] In the setting of percutaneous intervention, newer monitoring modalities such as the ecarin clotting time (ECT) have given preliminary promising results.[14] The half-life of bivalirudin ranges from 20 to 120 min, according to renal function.

Anticoagulation for intermittent claudication

The question of whether anticoagulants may be beneficial in patients with claudication has been recently addressed by the Cochrane Peripheral Vascular Diseases Review Group.[15] Thirteen trials were initially considered eligible for inclusion in the review: two studies evaluated oral anticoagulants, five evaluated standard heparin, and six evaluated LMWHs. Only three studies (two evaluating oral anticoagulants, one evaluating heparin) met the high-quality methodological inclusion criteria and were included in the primary analysis. Four other studies were included in the sensitivity analysis. The authors concluded that neither heparin, nor LMWHs, nor oral anticoagulants were beneficial in patients with intermittent claudication.

Anticoagulation during percutaneous transluminal angioplasty or stenting

As with percutaneous coronary intervention (PCI), the use of antithrombotic therapy in the setting of peripheral angioplasty and stenting relies on a balance between the reduction of ischemic complications and the bleeding risk. The endovascular treatment of peripheral disease has many similarities to PCI: namely, the basic equipment, the nature of the atherosclerotic disease, and the complications that may occur, both in the short term (e.g. dissection, abrupt vessel closure, thrombosis, distal embolization) and in the long term (e.g. restenosis, late occlusion). With respect to access-site-related complications, similarities between PCI and PTA include a femoral approach and similar sheath size. The higher likelihood of atherosclerotic disease of the common femoral artery may be a source of increased local complications in patients undergoing PTA, although no comparative studies have been performed.

The evidence available on adjunctive pharmacological treatment for PTA is far less solid than for PCI. One reason for this observation is the lack of surrogate markers of clinical outcome, such as creatine kinase-MB or troponin, which allow for a more precise assessment of antithrombotic drug efficacy. Furthermore, the extrapolation of data from PCI trials to the peripheral vasculature is problematic due to incomparable end points. While PCI trials have focused on death, myocardial infarction, or the need for revascularization, PAD intervention studies have mainly addressed patency rates and limb salvage. Platelet activation, adhesion, and aggregation are pivotal mechanisms of thrombus formation and vessel occlusion in both the coronary and peripheral vasculature. Although the importance of adequate antithrombotic therapy for successful PTA is evident, the optimal regimen still needs to be determined.

Unfractionated heparin

Since the beginning of coronary and peripheral intervention, UFH has been the anticoagulant of choice. Although, as previously described, its effect is largely unpredictable due to poor and markedly variable bioavailability, this limitation is probably of minor importance in the angiography suite since the level of anticoagulation is easily monitored using ACT. Whereas data in the coronary literature regarding the optimal level of periprocedural anticoagulation are limited and the topic is controversial, virtually no study has addressed the optimal level of anticoagulation for peripheral interventions. The impact on PTA results of other potential drawbacks of UFH (see Table 8.1), such as its proaggregatory effect and inability to inactivate clot-bound thrombin, is unknown. With respect to safety, a recent series examining bleeding complications following heparin-based PTA found a major bleeding rate of 4.6% among 213 consecutive patients.[16]

Low-molecular-weight heparin and bivalirudin

It is currently a source of debate whether UFH remains the anticoagulant of choice for both coronary and peripheral interventions. Potential alternatives include LMWH and the direct thrombin inhibitor bivalirudin. From a cost perspective, UFH is far less expensive than its competitors. Nevertheless, as previously described, LMWH has several potential advantages compared with UFH, including a predictable anticoagulant effect with no need for monitoring (see Table 8.1). Furthermore, LMWH has a higher ratio of factor Xa to thrombin inhibition, leading to inhibition of both thrombin generation and thrombin activity. To our knowledge, safety and efficacy of UFH and LMWH have not been compared in the setting of peripheral interventions.

Recently, the direct thrombin inhibitor bivalirudin has gained attention as an anticoagulant for PCI and PTA. The advantages of direct thrombin inhibitors over UFH include a more specific and potent inhibition of thrombin, acting independently from antithrombin and other endogenous factors (see Table 8.1). Unlike UFH, direct thrombin inhibitors are able to inhibit clot-bound thrombin and produce a more stable level of anticoagulation over time. Bivalirudin is more expensive than LMWH. In the coronary circulations, the benefit of these agents for the medical management of acute coronary syndromes over UFH has been only marginal and these agents have never found broad applications. More promising are the results in PCI with a large-scale clinical trial showing comparable efficacy and improved safety in patients treated with bivalirudin and provisional glycoprotein IIb/IIIa receptor inhibitor compared with UFH and planned glycoprotein IIb/IIIa receptor inhibitors.[17]

Preliminary data on bivalirudin-based anticoagulation during PTA appear encouraging. A single-center experience reported only two major bleeding complications (4.2%) among 48 consecutive patients undergoing lower extremity intervention.[18] Similarly, a retrospective analysis of 180 iliac and 75 renal revascularization procedures described a major or minor bleeding rate of 3.9%.[19] A multicenter registry of bivalirudin in peripheral intervention is ongoing. Randomized trials comparing the safety and efficacy of bivalirudin, LMWH, and UFH in the setting of PTA are warranted.

Monitoring and neutralization of anticoagulation during percutaneous interventions

Unfractionated heparin is widely used and offers several advantages as an antithrombotic regimen in the setting of percutaneous intervention. Measurements of ACT allow a precise and easy bedside monitoring of its antithrombotic activity, which, if needed, can be immediately reversed by protamine sulfate. Despite large experience in the use of UFH in the setting of PCI, the optimal dose of in-laboratory UFH for this indication still needs validation. The same is true for UFH-based anticoagulation in the setting of

PTA. To date, there is no rapid bedside assessment of LMWH antithrombotic activity, although this strategy is being explored. As previously mentioned, LMWH has little effect on aPTT and ACT, and the measurement of anti-Xa activity is cumbersome while being only a surrogate of potency. Moreover, LMWH's antithrombotic effect cannot be completely reversed with protamine. In fact, although protamine sulfate neutralizes the antithrombin activity of LMWH, it only partially reverses its anti-factor Xa activity.[20] Conversely, the antithrombotic effect of direct thrombin inhibitors may be assessed with aPTT or newer modalities such as ECT. Direct thrombin inhibitors also do not have a reversal agent. An advantage of bivalirudin over LMWH in the angiography suite is the shorter half-life.

Acute thromboembolic occlusion

In the setting of acute thromboembolic occlusion, the role of antithrombotic agents has not been established in clinical trials. The value of heparin treatment remains uncertain, but in the setting of urgent vascular surgery most investigators do administer heparin and continue the treatment throughout the perioperative period. If revascularization is delayed, heparin treatment may prevent or limit thrombotic propagation from the site of occlusion. The major role for anticoagulant therapy after embolization is to prevent embolic recurrence. Evidence available from retrospective, nonrandomized studies suggests that anticoagulant therapy with heparin or oral anticoagulants reduces the frequency of recurrence by approximately 75% compared with no therapy at the cost of higher incidence of wound complications, particularly hematomas.[21,22] Close monitoring and appropriate control of heparin given continuously after vascular operations may minimize bleeding complications. Other investigators have noted no reductions in recurrent emboli and mortality with postoperative heparin treatment.[23] To determine whether the benefits of postoperative anticoagulant therapy outweigh the risks, a randomized trial is necessary. The value of thrombolytic therapy in the setting of acute arterial occlusion is discussed in Chapter 7.

Anticoagulation in the setting of peripheral arterial bypass surgery

Intraoperative anticoagulation

Unfractionated heparin, usually administered at cross-clamps, remains the anticoagulant of choice during vascular surgery. The best route of administration (regional vs systemic) and optimal doses are unknown, and the issue of reversing or not reversing heparin by protamine sulfate following surgery has not been established.[24] The use of LMWH compared with UFH for intraoperative anticoagulation during infrainguinal bypass surgery has been investigated in three randomized clinical trials. Enoxaparin was compared with UFH in a multicenter trial enrolling 201 patients.[25] The drug was administered during surgery and for 10 days postoperatively. Graft thrombosis occurred in 8% of patients randomly assigned to receive LMWH and in 22% of those treated with UFH ($p = 0.009$). No difference in bleeding complications was observed. Limitations of the study included the short follow-up period (10 days) and the unusually high rate of graft thrombosis in the UFH group. In the second study 18 patients undergoing infrainguinal bypass were randomly assigned to dalteparin or UFH.[26] Two early graft occlusions occurred in each group, and one bleeding complication occurred in the UFH group.

The third study, recently published, adds important information on periprocedural safety and efficacy of LMWH for vascular surgery.[27] The study was an open label, prospective, randomized trial, carried out by 20 Swedish centers and enrolled patients undergoing peripheral vascular surgery with the exception of carotid endarterectomy. Of the 849 patients included, 817 were followed up to 30 days. Enoxaparin (40 mg) or UFH (5000 IU) were given intravenously immediately before clamping. The same formulation in diluted form was used for vascular rinsing. The overall mortality rate at 30 days was 2.7%, with no difference between groups. No differences were observed in graft patency rates. Median blood loss was 350 mL in the LMWH group and 425 mL in the UFH group ($p = 0.02$). The authors concluded that LMWH was comparable to UFH during peripheral vascular reconstruction in terms of graft patency, operative blood loss, and hemorrhagic complications.

Overall, LMWH and UFH appear to have similar safety and efficacy profiles in the setting of perioperative anticoagulation. Drawbacks of LMWH use in this setting include its longer half-life and the absence of an efficacious antagonist. The lack of reversibility is of particular concern for procedures such as aortic revascularization and for bypass procedures performed with prosthetic materials which are prone to suture hole bleeding. Although the optimal length of perioperative heparinization is unknown, most surgeons do not routinely use therapeutic heparin or other anticoagulants beyond the intraoperative period.

Secondary prevention following surgery: antiplatelet agents or anticoagulants?

As with PTA, the risks and benefits of antiplatelet therapy or anticoagulation following peripheral bypass surgery require careful evaluation. Compared with endovascular therapy, surgery is associated with an increased risk of cardiovascular events. More evidence is available on the impact of antithrombotic therapy following peripheral bypass surgery than post-PTA. An analysis of 10 randomized trials detected an overall 24% event reduction among patients undergoing lower limb bypass who were treated with antiplatelet agents compared with placebo.[28] A meta-analysis by the Antiplatelet Trialists' Collaboration demonstrated that, among around 2000 patients undergoing peripheral bypass surgery, there was an approximately 40% reduction in graft occlusion in patients treated with antiplatelet agents (mostly aspirin).[29] A placebo-controlled study similarly showed improved patency with ticlopidine.[30] The value of dual antiplatelet therapy in this setting is being investigated in the CASPAR (Clopidogrel and Acetylsalicylic Acid in Bypass Surgery for Peripheral Arterial Disease) trial.

The benefit of antithrombotic therapy following lower extremity bypass surgery has been recently addressed in a meta-analysis.[31] Only three randomized trials, for a total of 334 patients, compared oral anticoagulation and placebo.[32–34] At a follow-up, ranging between 12 and 120 months, oral anticoagulation halved the incidence of graft occlusion (OR 0.54, 95% CI 0.28–1.04) compared with placebo. The results did not reach statistical significance due to the limited sample size. The first of the three studies was a randomized, prospective trial of 88 patients with reversed saphenous vein femoropopliteal bypasses and demonstrated a significant reduction in bypass occlusion associated with anticoagulation (18% vs 37% among controls; $p < 0.03$) after a mean follow-up of 30 months.[32] Of concern is that 12% of the patients in the active treatment arm had to discontinue anticoagulant therapy because of major bleeding. In the second study, 116 patients undergoing vein and prosthetic lower-extremity bypasses were randomly assigned to oral anticoagulation or no anticoagulant therapy and followed for up to 3 years.[33] There were no statistically significant differences in patency, limb salvage, or survival rates between control and oral anticoagulant-treated groups. Bleeding complications were more frequent in treated patients and included 5% serious or life-threatening bleedings. Another study of 130 patients demonstrated significant improvement in graft patency among patients treated with oral anticoagulants in comparison with controls.[34] This study had a 10-year follow-up. Arterial graft patency and survival were significantly improved in patients treated with oral anticoagulants.

The effect of the combination of warfarin and aspirin vs aspirin alone on the patency of infrainguinal vein bypass grafts among patients deemed to be at high risk for graft failure was evaluated in a single-center, randomized clinical trial of 56 patients.[35] Aspirin dosage was 325 mg/day, and warfarin was given to maintain the international normalized ratio (INR) between 2 and 3. Patients assigned to warfarin received heparin anticoagulation postoperatively, which was then converted to warfarin. The high-risk inclusion criteria were marginal quality vein, poor arterial runoff, and previously failed bypass. Bypass to the tibial arteries was performed in 90% of patients. The 3-year primary patency

111

rate (78% vs 41%) and the limb salvage rate were significantly higher in those patients randomly assigned to warfarin. Despite the higher incidence of hematomas in the warfarin group (35% vs 3.7%), the overall complication rate did not differ between groups. Although a benefit from the routine use of oral anticoagulation after uncomplicated femorotibial bypass procedures has not been demonstrated, patients considered to be at high risk for thrombosis might be considered for postoperative anticoagulation.

The effect of oral anticoagulation compared with aspirin after infrainguinal bypass surgery was evaluated in a multicenter randomized clinical trial enrolling a total of 2690 patients, the Dutch Bypass Oral anticoagulants or Aspirin (BOA) study.[36] Patients were randomly assigned to receive either oral anticoagulation (target INR 3.0–4.5; $n = 1339$) or aspirin (80 mg daily, $n = 1351$). At a mean of 21 months' follow-up, there were 308 graft occlusions in the oral anticoagulation group compared with 322 graft occlusions with aspirin (hazard ratio 0.95, 95% CI 0.82–1.11), suggesting no overall benefit from either treatment. Subgroup analysis suggested that oral anticoagulants were beneficial in patients with vein grafts (hazard ratio 0.69, 95% CI 0.54–0.88), whereas aspirin had better results for non-venous grafts (hazard ratio 1.26, 95% CI 1.03–1.55). The composite outcome of vascular death, myocardial infarction, stroke, or amputation occurred 248 times in the oral anticoagulants group and 275 times in the aspirin group (hazard ratio 0.89, 95% CI 0.75–1.06). Patients treated with oral anticoagulants had more major bleeding episodes than those treated with aspirin (108 vs 56; hazard ratio 1.96, 95% CI 1.42–2.71). Although the overall results do not support routine use of oral anticoagulation after infrainguinal bypass, the results of the subgroup analysis suggested that the antithrombotic strategy should be tailored according to graft type.

Low-intensity oral anticoagulant therapy (INR 1.5–2) combined with low-dose aspirin therapy (80–325 mg) is an attractive antithrombotic regimen. Lower doses of these combined agents might offer superior antithrombotic effectiveness while minimizing hemorrhagic side effects. This combination was evaluated in a multicenter randomized trial conducted in Department of Veterans Affairs hospitals.[37] A total of 831 patients who underwent peripheral arterial bypass surgery were compared in a long-term treatment program of warfarin (target INR 1.4–2.8) plus aspirin (325 mg/day) vs aspirin alone. The primary end point was bypass patency, and mortality and morbidity were the secondary end points. After a mean follow-up of 3 years, the mortality was 31.8% in the combination group and 23.0% in the aspirin group (risk ratio 1.41, 95% CI 1.09–1.84, $p = 0.0001$). Major hemorrhagic events occurred significantly more frequently in the combination group. In the prosthetic bypass group, there was no significant difference in patency rate in the 8-mm bypass subgroup, but there was a significant difference in patency rate in the 6-mm bypass subgroup (femoropopliteal, 71.4% in the combination group vs 57.9%

in the aspirin group, $p = 0.02$). In the vein bypass group, patency rate was unaffected (75.3% in the combination group vs 74.9% in the aspirin group). Therefore, the advantage of oral anticoagulation among patients treated with vein graft observed in a subgroup analysis of the BOA trial[37] could not be reproduced. The authors concluded that long-term administration of warfarin in combination with aspirin was limited to few selected indications for improvement of bypass patency and that it was associated with an increased risk of morbidity and mortality. Currently, the American College of Chest Physicians (ACCP) recommends the combination of warfarin (INR 2–3) and aspirin (80–325 mg) for patients deemed to be at high risk of graft failure.[24]

The experience with prolonged anticoagulation following vascular surgery with non-coumarin derivatives has been limited. In a study of 200 patients, LMWH administered for 3 months was compared with aspirin and dipyridamole in patients undergoing femoropopliteal bypass.[38] Not only was patency significantly better with LMWH treatment but also the effects persisted and became more evident with time. Although these observations are of interest, long-term LMWH therapy does not appear to be a viable option due to cumbersome administration and side effects. The oral thrombin inhibitor ximelagatran, which has recently demonstrated safety and efficacy in thromboembolic prevention in patients with atrial fibrillation, has not yet been tested in the peripheral vasculature. As in other fields of cardiovascular medicine, it is conceivable that oral anticoagulants administered in fixed dose with no need for monitoring of the anticoagulation level may replace warfarin in the future.

ACCP recommendations on anticoagulation for peripheral arterial disease

The ACCP recommends systemic anticoagulation with UFH for patients with acute treatment of thromboembolic events involving the peripheral vasculature to prevent proximal/distal thrombotic propagation.[24] Heparin should be followed by oral anticoagulation to prevent recurrent embolism in patients undergoing thromboembolectomy. Intra-arterial thrombolytic therapy should be considered in patients with short-term (<14 days) thrombotic or embolic occlusive disease.

All patients following peripheral bypass surgery should receive long-term antiplatelet therapy for secondary cardiovascular prevention. Long-term oral anticoagulation with warfarin with or without aspirin may be considered in selected patients after infrainguinal bypass and other vascular reconstructions. For patients undergoing infrainguinal bypass deemed at high risk of graft thrombosis, a combination treatment of warfarin and aspirin is recommended. During major vascular reconstructive surgery, systemic anticoagulation with UFH should be administered at the time of cross-clamps.

Conclusions

The most frequent use of anticoagulants in patients with PAD is in the setting of percutaneous or surgical revascularization. The most widely used and by far less-expensive agent is UFH. Although this agent has several pharmacokinetic and pharmacodynamic limitations, it is unclear whether these properties play a role in the setting of brief periprocedural anticoagulation. Although of potential interest, alternative anticoagulants such as LMWH or the direct thrombin inhibitor bivalirudin have not been adequately tested in the setting of percutaneous or surgical vascular procedures. Overall, long-term oral anticoagulation does not appear to confer additional long-term benefits compared to aspirin among patients who have undergone vascular surgery. However, in selected patients oral anticoagulation may be considered. In subjects deemed to be at high risk for graft occlusion, a combination of low-dose aspirin and oral anticoagulation appears to be a valid option. The oral thrombin inhibitors have not been tested in the peripheral vasculature. As in other fields of cardiovascular medicine, it is conceivable that oral anticoagulants administered in fixed dose with no need for monitoring of the anticoagulation level may replace warfarin in the future.

Key points
- UFH is still the anticoagulant of choice for percutaneous or surgical vascular procedures.
- LMWH and bivalirudin are attractive alternatives to UFH but have not been adequately studied.
- Overall, long-term oral anticoagulation is of no additional benefit compared to aspirin among patients who have undergone surgery.
- In selected high-risk patients following peripheral bypass surgery, long-term oral anticoagulation with or without aspirin may be considered.
- In the future, oral anticoagulants administered in fixed dose with no need for monitoring of the anticoagulation level (e.g. ximelagatran) may replace warfarin.

References

1. Roffi M, Topol EJ. Anticoagulant therapy in unstable angina. In: Topol EJ, ed. Textbook of cardiovascular medicine update series, Vol. 3. New York: Lippincott, Williams & Wilkins; 2000:1–11.

2. Fenton JW 2nd, Ofosu FA, Moon DG, Maraganore JM. Thrombin structure and function: why thrombin is the primary target for antithrombotics. Blood Coagul Fibrinolysis 1991;2:69–75.

3. Verstraete M. Direct thrombin inhibitors: appraisal of the antithrombotic/ hemorrhagic balance. Thromb Haemost 1997;78:357–63.

4. Stubbs MT, Bode W. A player of many parts: the spotlight falls on thrombin's structure. Thromb Res 1993;69:1–58.

5. Hirsh J, Raschke R, Warkentin TE, et al. Heparin: mechanism of action, pharmacokinetics, dosing considerations, monitoring, efficacy, and safety. Chest 1995;108:258S–275S.

6. Weitz JI, Hudoba M, Massel D, Maraganore J, Hirsh J. Clot-bound thrombin is protected from inhibition by heparin-antithrombin III but is susceptible to inactivation by antithrombin III-independent inhibitors. J Clin Invest 1990;86:385–91.

7. Hirsh J, Weitz J. Antithrombin therapy. In: Califf R, Braunwald E, eds. Atlas of heart disease, Vol. VIII. Philadelphia: Current Medicine; 1996:9.1.

8. Brieger DB, Mak KH, Kottke-Marchant K, Topol EJ. Heparin-induced thrombocytopenia. J Am Coll Cardiol 1998;31:1449–59.

9. Mammen EF, Arcelus J, Messmore H, et al. Clinical differentiation of low molecular weight heparins. Semin Thromb Hemost 1999;25:135–44.

10. Warkentin TE, Levine MN, Hirsh J, et al. Heparin-induced thrombocytopenia in patients treated with low-molecular-weight heparin or unfractionated heparin. N Engl J Med 1995;332:1330–5.

11. Rao AK, Sun L, Chesebro JH, et al. Distinct effects of recombinant desulfatohirudin (Revasc) and heparin on plasma levels of fibrinopeptide A and prothrombin fragment F1.2 in unstable angina. A multicenter trial. Circulation 1996;94:2389–95.

12. Laposata M, Green D, Van Cott EM, et al. College of American Pathologists Conference XXXI on laboratory monitoring of anticoagulant therapy: the clinical use and laboratory monitoring of low-molecular-weight heparin, danaparoid, hirudin and related compounds, and argatroban. Arch Pathol Lab Med 1998;122:799–807.

13. Zoldhelyi P, Webster MW, Fuster V, et al. Recombinant hirudin in patients with chronic, stable coronary artery disease. Safety, half-life, and effect on coagulation parameters. Circulation 1993;88:2015–22.

14. Cho L, Kottke-Marchant K, Lincoff AM, et al. Correlation of point-of-care ecarin clotting time versus activated clotting time with bivalirudin concentrations. Am J Cardiol 2003;91:1110–13.

15. Cosmi B, Conti E, Coccheri S. Anticoagulants (heparin, low molecular weight heparin and oral anticoagulants) for intermittent claudication. Cochrane Database Syst Rev 2001:CD001999.

16. Shammas NW, Lemke JH, Dippel EJ, et al. In-hospital complications of peripheral vascular interventions using unfractionated heparin as the primary anticoagulant. J Invasive Cardiol 2003;15:242–6.

17. Lincoff AM, Bittl JA, Harrington RA, et al. Bivalirudin and provisional glycoprotein IIb/IIIa blockade compared with heparin and planned glycoprotein IIb/IIIa blockade during percutaneous coronary intervention: REPLACE–2 randomized trial. JAMA 2003;289:853–63.

18. Shammas NW, Lemke JH, Dippel EJ, et al. Bivalirudin in peripheral vascular interventions: a single center experience. J Invasive Cardiol 2003;15:401–4.

19. Allie DE, Lirtzman MD, Wyatt CH, et al. Bivalirudin as a foundation anticoagulant in peripheral vascular disease: a safe and feasible alternative for renal and iliac interventions. J Invasive Cardiol 2003;15:334–42.

20. Wolzt M, Weltermann A, Nieszpaur-Los M, et al. Studies on the neutralizing effects of protamine on unfractionated and low molecular weight heparin (Fragmin) at the site of activation of the coagulation system in man. Thromb Haemost 1995;73:439–43.

21. Holm J, Schersten T. Anticoagulant treatment during and after embolectomy. Acta Chir Scand 1972;138:683–7.

22. Elliott JP Jr, Hageman JH, Szilagyi E, et al. Arterial embolization: problems of source, multiplicity, recurrence, and delayed treatment. Surgery 1980;88:833–45.

23. Silvers LW, Royster TS, Mulcare RJ. Peripheral arterial emboli and factors in their recurrence rate. Ann Surg 1980;192:232–6.

24. Jackson MR, Clagett GP. Antithrombotic therapy in peripheral arterial occlusive disease. Chest 2001;119:283S–299S.

25. Samama CM, Gigou F, Ill P. Low-molecular-weight heparin vs. unfractionated heparin in femorodistal reconstructive surgery: a multicenter open randomized study. Enoxart Study Group. Ann Vasc Surg 1995;9 Suppl:S45–53.

26. Swedenborg J, Nydahl S, Egberg N. Low molecular mass heparin instead of unfractionated heparin during infrainguinal bypass surgery. Eur J Vasc Endovasc Surg 1996;11:59–64.

27. Norgren L. Can low molecular weight heparin replace unfractionated heparin during peripheral arterial reconstruction? An open label prospective randomized controlled trial. J Vasc Surg 2004;39:977–84.

28. Robless P, Mikhailidis DP, Stansby G. Systematic review of antiplatelet therapy for the prevention of myocardial infarction, stroke or vascular death in patients with peripheral vascular disease. Br J Surg 2001;88:787–800.

29. Collaborative overview of randomised trials of antiplatelet therapy – II: Maintenance of vascular graft or arterial patency by antiplatelet therapy. Antiplatelet Trialists' Collaboration. BMJ 1994;308:159–68.

30. Becquemin JP. Effect of ticlopidine on the long-term patency of saphenous-vein bypass grafts in the legs. Etude de la Ticlopidine apres Pontage Femoro-Poplite and the Association Universitaire de Recherche en Chirurgie. N Engl J Med 1997;337:1726–31.

31. Collins TC, Souchek J, Beyth RJ. Benefits of antithrombotic therapy after infrainguinal bypass grafting: a meta-analysis. Am J Med 2004;117:93–9.

32. Kretschmer G, Wenzl E, Piza F, et al. The influence of anticoagulant treatment on the probability of function in femoropopliteal vein bypass surgery: analysis of a clinical series (1970 to 1985) and interim evaluation of a controlled clinical trial. Surgery 1987;102:453–9.

33. Arfvidsson B, Lundgren F, Drott C, Schersten T, Lundholm K. Influence of coumarin treatment on patency and limb salvage after peripheral arterial reconstructive surgery. Am J Surg 1990;159:556–60.

34. Kretschmer G, Herbst F, Prager M, et al. A decade of oral anticoagulant treatment to maintain autologous vein grafts for femoropopliteal atherosclerosis. Arch Surg 1992;127:1112–15.

35. Sarac TP, Huber TS, Back MR, et al. Warfarin improves the outcome of infrainguinal vein bypass grafting at high risk for failure. J Vasc Surg 1998;28:446–57.

36. Efficacy of oral anticoagulants compared with aspirin after infrainguinal bypass surgery (the Dutch Bypass Oral anticoagulants or Aspirin study): a randomised trial. Lancet 2000;355:346–51.

37. Johnson WC, Williford WO. Benefits, morbidity, and mortality associated with long-term administration of oral anticoagulant therapy to patients with peripheral arterial bypass procedures: a prospective randomized study. J Vasc Surg 2002;35:413–21.

38. Edmondson RA, Cohen AT, Das SK, Wagner MB, Kakkar VV. Low-molecular weight heparin versus aspirin and dipyridamole after femoropopliteal bypass grafting. Lancet 1994;344:914–18.

39. Lauer MA, Lincoff AM. Parenteral direct antithrombins. In: Uprichard ACG, Gallagher KP, eds. Handbook of experimental pharmacology. Volume on antithrombins. New York: Springer-Verlag; 1998.

9. MISCELLANEOUS AGENTS

Juhana Karha and Samir R Kapadia

Naftidrofuryl

Naftidrofuryl has been used in Europe since the 1970s in the treatment of symptomatic peripheral arterial disease (intermittent claudication). It is not clear which mechanism is responsible for the benefit that has been observed with its clinical use. Naftidrofuryl acts via succinodehydrogenase to improve aerobic glucose metabolism with corresponding reduction in lactate levels. It also blocks serotonin-2 receptors (5-hydroxytryptamine-2 [5-HT2]) found on the vascular wall smooth muscle cells, and thus limits ischemic injury to endothelium and decreases serotonin-mediated vasoconstriction and smooth muscle cell proliferation.[1] The 5-HT2 receptors are also found on platelets and naftidrofuryl may potentially act via inhibiting platelet aggregation. Moreover, naftidrofuryl also reduces erythrocyte aggregability and rigidity.

Initial studies recording peripheral transcutaneous oxygen pressure showed positive results, including in areas of ischemia and ulceration, prompting clinical evaluation.[2,3] Notably, this increase in oxygen tension seemed to be independent of the arterial blood flow. In animal experiments, a single dose of intra-arterial (or intramuscular) naftidrofuryl caused marked vasodilation of a dog femoral artery.[4,5] Likewise, among healthy human volunteers, naftidrofuryl administration resulted in lower-extremity arterial vasodilation, paving the way for clinical trials in patients with peripheral arterial disease.[6]

In a study by Trubestein et al, 104 patients with angiographically confirmed lower-extremity arterial disease were randomized to receive oral naftidrofuryl (200 mg three times daily) vs placebo.[7] After a 4-week run-in phase to ensure stable disease profile, patients underwent a 12-week treatment phase. Both groups achieved increases in the pain-free walking distance (PFWD), with significantly greater increase in the treatment group (improvement from 137 m to 230 m vs 135 m to 171 m in the placebo group, $p < 0.05$), (Table 9.1). Notably, no difference was detected between the two groups in the maximal walking distance (MWD) following therapy. Adhoute et al studied 118 Fontaine classification II patients following a 30-day run-in period.[8] They were randomized to oral naftidrofuryl (200 mg three times daily) vs placebo for 6 months. The PFWD increased in both groups, from a baseline of 215 m, to

Table 9.1 Summary of Clinical Trials

Drug/study	Number of patients	Percent improvement in PFWD	p-value
Naftidrofuryl			
Trubestein[7]	104	68	<0.05
Adhoute[8]	118	93	<0.05
Kriessmann[9]	136	78	<0.05
L-arginine			
Boger[23]	39	230	<0.05
Maxwell[26]	41	66	<0.05
Prostaglandins			
Boger[23]	39	209	<0.05
Scheffler[28]	44	604	<0.05
Diehm[29]	213	104	<0.05
Mangiafico[30]	42	87	<0.05
Lievre[33]	162	129	<0.05
Lievre[34]	422	82	<0.05

416 m and 313 m for the treatment and placebo groups, respectively, with $p < 0.05$. In another randomized study, by Kriessmann and Neiss, 136 patients with claudication (Fontaine class II) received oral naftidrofuryl (316.5 mg twice daily) vs placebo, and derived treatment benefit as assessed by PFWD after a 12-week course: 208 m vs 163 m (up from baseline 117 m vs 121 m) in the treatment vs placebo groups, respectively, $p < 0.05$.[9] In another 6-month randomized study by Adhoute et al, a 316.5 mg twice-daily oral naftidrofuryl regimen was superior to placebo, as measured by both PFWD and MWD.[10] The final pain-free and maximal walking distances were 351 m vs 287 m, $p < 0.05$, and 469 m vs 337 m, $p < 0.01$, for the treatment and placebo groups, respectively. Importantly, fewer patients in the naftidrofuryl arm required surgical revascularization procedures during the study period compared to patients in the placebo group: 12% vs 30% (p-value not provided). A meta-analysis of these four trials[7–10] reveals a 3-month increase in PFWD of 96 m vs 41 m for naftidrofuryl vs placebo-treated patients, respectively.[11] The most promising results were noted in patients with longer initial walking distances.

De Backer and colleagues attempted to perform a meta-analysis[12] on nine placebo-controlled randomized trials that evaluated the use of naftidrofuryl in peripheral arterial disease.[8–10,13–18] In the authors' assessment, three trials reported variability of the results in insufficient detail and lacked internal validity.[13,14,16] Among the remaining six trials,[8–10,15,17,18] including three out of the four included in the meta-analysis discussed above,[11] the authors felt that excessive intra- and inter-trial variation precluded a reliable meta-analysis.[12] However, despite these inconsistencies, five out of the six trials documented statistically significant improvement in PFWD when compared to placebo. These mean increases ranged between 7 and 103 m over placebo. As with any series of small published trials, the possibility of publication bias cannot be excluded.

The data for the use of naftidrofuryl in more severe peripheral arterial disease is even sparser. Moody et al randomized 188 patients with severe intermittent claudication (mean baseline PFWD of 60 m) to naftidrofuryl vs placebo for 6 months and failed to document a difference in the PFWD.[13] However, oral naftidrofuryl has been promising in healing vascular ulcers in few patients following 2–3 months of therapy compared to placebo.[3,19]

The currently available data regarding naftidrofuryl efficacy have several limitations. The major limitation has been the small number of patients in each study. The meta-analyses have been difficult to interpret due to variations in study designs and probable selection bias. Further, some trials enrolling patients with intermittent claudication have used crossover design, which can be suboptimal given the progressive nature of peripheral arterial disease in some patients.[14,15] Other trials have not utilized a proper placebo run-in period.[16,17,20] In sum, the data for the efficacy of this medication in treating peripheral vascular disease are inconclusive at best.

The side-effect profile of naftidrofuryl is rather benign. Gastrointestinal distress is the most common side effect and led to withdrawal from the trial in 1.2% of patients (compared to 0.95% with placebo).[11] More rare side effects that have been reported include flushing, hepatic necrosis, and esophageal ulceration. Following a number of cases of severe cardiac and neurological toxicity in patients who received intravenous bolus administration of naftidrofuryl, the intravenous formulation was pulled from the European market in 1995.

Naftidrofuryl is stored in fatty tissue and metabolized by plasma pseudocholinesterases. The plasma elimination half-life is up to 2 hours, thus requiring three-times daily administration. The common dosage is 100–200 mg three times daily. Dose reduction may be required in elderly patients due to longer plasma elimination half-life.

In conclusion, the data examining the possible clinical benefit with naftidrofuryl in peripheral arterial disease are sparse and no recent trials have been performed. No definitive evidence exists that naftidrofuryl offers a meaningful benefit over placebo based on these studies. However, the data are suggestive that naftidrofuryl may offer a small benefit. In the current American practice, naftidrofuryl is not used in the treatment of peripheral arterial disease, but it has been used in Europe.

L-arginine

A putative mechanism contributing to intermittent claudication is impaired vasodilation. Atherosclerosis is characterized by impaired endothelium-dependent vasodilation, a process in which nitric oxide plays a key role. Patients with peripheral arterial disease experience progressive reduction in urinary nitrate and cGMP excretion, both markers of active nitric oxide metabolism.[21] This may be caused by the accumulation of asymmetric dimethylarginine (ADMA), an endogenous nitric oxide synthase inhibitor.[21] Nitric oxide (NO) formed by the vessel wall mediates endothelium-dependent vasodilation, and thus has been the focus of several investigators in the field. L-arginine serves as the precursor amino acid in the formation of nitric oxide. Animal studies have demonstrated that administration of exogenous L-arginine improves the endothelium-dependent vasodilation.[22] Likewise, administration of L-arginine has been noted to increase NO production and endothelium-dependent vasodilation among patients with atherosclerotic vascular disease.[23,24] Other candidate mechanisms for the beneficial effect of L-arginine are inhibition of monocyte adhesion to the vascular endothelium, antioxidant properties, and analgesic effect.

Intravenous L-arginine, at the dose of 8 g twice daily for 3 weeks, was shown to increase PFWD and MWD among 39 randomized patients with peripheral arterial disease compared to no drug therapy (no placebo group): 230% improvement (52 m to 147 m) vs no change, $p < 0.05$, and 155% improvement (93 m to 216 m) vs no change, $p < 0.05$, respectively.[23] The medication was well tolerated, with one subject experiencing mild skin rash. In the same study, femoral artery endothelium-dependent vasodilation, as assessed by ultrasonography, was increased by administration of L-arginine. Consistent with these results, L-arginine also improved pain, as assessed subjectively by the patients. It is also notable that the patients receiving L-arginine had higher urinary excretion rates of nitrates and cGMP. The ratio of plasma L-arginine to dimethylarginine was also increased among the patients receiving the medication.[23]

A positron emission tomography study by Schellong et al documented an increase in the tissue-level perfusion by measuring calf muscle blood flow of patients with peripheral arterial disease receiving intravenous L-arginine.[25] The increase in muscle perfusion coincided with a parallel increase in the plasma cGMP level. One drawback with L-arginine is the need to take large doses of the medication (16 g/day).

Minimal data are available for the use of oral L-arginine. Maxwell and colleagues randomized 41 patients with peripheral arterial disease in a double-blind, placebo-controlled fashion to L-arginine-enriched food bars (one or two bars per day) for 2 weeks.[26] Patients who consumed 2 bars daily improved their PFWD by 66% (p <0.05 compared to baseline; no improvements among patients receiving placebo or consuming 1 bar per day). Xerostomia occurred in two subjects, and there were no other significant side effects.

In total, the evidence for symptomatic benefit of L-arginine in peripheral arterial disease is scant, but there is some suggestion that it may offer a modest benefit.

Prostaglandins

Prostaglandin E_1 (PGE_1) activates prostacyclin receptors, and thus mediates endothelium-independent vasodilatation. Prostaglandin E_1 also inhibits platelet aggregation. Prostaglandins have been evaluated for peripheral arterial disease in a number of clinical trials. In a 1560-patient randomized multicenter trial studying chronic critical limb ischemia, 60 µg of daily intravenous open-label alprostadil (PGE_1) for the duration hospital stay (up to 28 days) was compared with no therapy.[27] The patients in the prostaglandin group had a higher rate of resolution of ischemia (p <0.001), but there was no difference in the rates of amputation or mortality. In another study by Boger et al, 39 patients with peripheral arterial disease were randomized to receive a 3-week course of PGE_1 (40 µg intravenously twice daily) vs L-arginine (see previous section on L-arginine) vs no therapy.[23] The prostaglandin therapy improved both the PFWD and the MWD by 209% and 144% compared to baseline, respectively, while patients receiving no therapy had no significant improvements in the walking distances (p <0.05 for PGE_1 vs placebo comparisons for both PFWD and MWD). Of note, these improvements were slightly smaller than those seen with L-arginine therapy (p = NS).

A study by Scheffler and colleagues randomized 44 patients with intermittent claudication, with all undergoing exercise training, to open-label prostaglandin PGE_1 (40 µg intravenously twice daily for 4 weeks) vs intravenous pentoxifylline vs no additional pharmacological therapy. The patients in the prostaglandin group had better relief of claudication compared to the other two groups.[28] The percentage increases in PFWD in the three groups were 604%, 105%, and 119%, for PGE_1, pentoxifylline, and no added therapy, respectively (p <0.05 for PGE_1 vs either of the other groups). A randomized, double-blind study of 213 patients with intermittent claudication revealed that an 8-week course of intravenous PGE_1 vs placebo improved PFWD by 104% at 3 months compared to baseline (placebo group with 63% improvement, p <0.05 for superior effect of PGE_1).[29] In this study, 13% vs 8% of the patients developed side effects, mainly at the infusion site, but importantly, there were no instances of hypotension. Another study by

Mangiafico et al also documented benefits with a 4-week course of daily intravenous PGE_1 (60 μg) in 42 patients with intermittent claudication (87% improvement over baseline in PFWD vs no improvement in the placebo group at the end of the 4-week treatment course).[30] This benefit persisted at 8 weeks after the last dose (57% vs no improvement).

The major limitation of intravenous PGE_1 is the cumbersome administration and the short half-life of the drug. To overcome this limitation, multiple strategies have been tested. Lipid-bound microsphere formulation may extend the half-life of the drug. In another blinded randomized study, a 4-week course of daily intravenous infusion of an acylated and esterified prodrug for PGE_1 (AS-013), incorporated into microspheres and activated by the endothelium in a hydrolysis step, improved MWD and PFWD and symptoms modestly over placebo in 80 patients with intermittent claudication.[31]

Prostaglandin I_2 (PGI_2) has a short half-life, and iloprost, a PGI_2 analogue, was developed to lengthen the half-life. It offers some improvement in amputation-free survival, along with pain relief and improved ulcer healing, in patients with severe peripheral arterial disease.[32] Beraprost is an oral PGI_2 (epoprostenol) analogue with a half-life of ~0.6 hours. In a double-blind study examining beraprost (Beraprost et Claudication Intermittente, BERCI), 164 patients with intermittent claudication were randomized to three beraprost doses (20 μg, 40 μg, and 60 μg three times daily) and to placebo for a total of 12 weeks.[33] The patients in the two lower beraprost dose groups had small improvements in PFWD, but interestingly, the highest beraprost dose did not improve PFWD. The percent PFWD improvements over baseline were 129%, 114%, and 51% for the three beraprost doses, respectively, and 58% for the placebo group. Despite these small benefits with the lower doses, 62% of the patients receiving beraprost developed side effects of headache, flushing, and gastrointestinal distress.[33] In a larger trial, 422 patients were randomized in a double-blinded fashion to receive beraprost 40 μg three times daily for 6 months vs placebo. The beraprost group experienced greater improvement in PFWD (81.5% vs 52.5%, $p = 0.001$) and less critical limb ischemia.[34] In this trial, a total of 17% of patients in the beraprost arm developed side effects of headache and flushing. A more recent and larger trial by Mohler and colleagues randomized 897 patients with intermittent claudication to beraprost 40 μg three times daily vs placebo.[35] There was no significant difference in MWD or PFWD between the groups after 3 and 6 months of treatment.

In summary, despite the encouraging initial results of prostaglandin use for intermittent claudication, the recent larger trial of the oral preparation does not support a more widespread clinical use.

Key points

- Although small studies have suggested some clinical benefit with naftidrofuryl in patients with moderate peripheral arterial disease, objective data are sparse and no recent randomized trials have been performed.
- The evidence for symptomatic benefit of L-arginine in patients with peripheral arterial disease is scant, but there is some suggestion that it may offer a modest benefit.
- Intravenous administration of prostaglandins has been associated with clinical benefits but their use is limited by cumbersome administration regimens and the short half-life of the drug.
- Oral prostaglandin preparations such as the PGI_2 analogue beraprost do not improve the symptoms of claudication.

References

1. Wiernsperger NF. Serotonin, 5-HT2 receptors, and their blockade by naftidrofuryl: a targeted therapy of vascular diseases. J Cardiovasc Pharmacol 1994;23(Suppl 3):S37–43.

2. Pointel JP, Thomas C, Mosnier M, et al. tcpO$_2$, arterial blood flow and lactate/pyruvate modifications induced by a single dose of naftidrofuryl IV during stage III lower-limb arteriopathies. Angiology 1986;37:647–53.

3. Kalis B. Assessment by transcutaneous PO$_2$ measurement of the treatment of venous ulcers with naftidrofuryl. J Mal Vasc 1984;9:133–6.

4. Moore N, Leclerc JL, Saligaut C, et al. [Comparative vasodilator action of 5 vasodilators: dihydroergotoxine, nicergoline, papaverine, naftidrofuryl and buflomedil on the femoral artery of the dog]. J Pharmacol 1982;13:423–30.

5. Luong TN, Depin JC. [Comparative study of femoral vasodilatator effects of naftidrofuryl and nicergoline on dog (author's translation)]. J Pharmacol 1981;12:263–75.

6. Gaylarde PM, Tan OT, Sarkany I. Blood flow changes with naftidrofuryl in systemic sclerosis and Raynaud's phenomenon. Br J Dermatol 1980;102:7–10.

7. Trubestein G, Bohme H, Heidrich H, et al. Naftidrofuryl in chronic arterial disease. Results of a controlled multicenter study. Angiology 1984;35:701–8.

8. Adhoute G, Bacourt F, Barral M, et al. Naftidrofuryl in chronic arterial disease. Results of a six month controlled multicenter study using Naftidrofuryl tablets 200 mg. Angiology 1986;37:160–7.

9. Kriessmann A, Neiss A. [Clinical effectiveness of naftidrofuryl in intermittent claudication]. Vasa Suppl 1988;24:27–32.

10. Adhoute G, Andreassian B, Boccalon H, et al. Treatment of stage II chronic arterial disease of the lower limbs with the serotonergic antagonist naftidrofuryl: results after 6 months of a controlled, multicenter study. J Cardiovasc Pharmacol 1990;16(Suppl)3:S75–80.

11. Lehert P, Riphagen FE, Gamand S. The effect of naftidrofuryl on intermittent claudication: a meta-analysis. J Cardiovasc Pharmacol 1990;16(Suppl)3:S81–6.

12. De Backer TL, Vander Stichele RH, Warie HH, Bogaert MG. Oral vasoactive medication in intermittent claudication: utile or futile? Eur J Clin Pharmacol 2000;56:199–206.

13. Moody AP, al-Khaffaf HS, Lehert P, et al. An evaluation of patients with severe intermittent claudication and the effect of treatment with naftidrofuryl. J Cardiovasc Pharmacol 1994;23(Suppl 3):S44–7.

14. Karnik R, Valentin A, Stollberger C, Slany J. Effects of naftidrofuryl in patients with intermittent claudication. Angiology 1988;39:234–40.

15. Pohle W, Hirche H, Barmeyer J, et al. [Double-blind study of naftidrofuryl-hydrogen oxalate in peripheral arterial occlusive disease]. Med Welt 1979;30:269–72.

16. Ruckley CV, Callam MJ, Ferrington CM, Prescott RJ. Naftidrofuryl for intermittent claudication: a double-blind controlled trial. Br Med J 1978;1:622.

17. Clyne CA, Galland RB, Fox MJ, et al. A controlled trial of naftidrofuryl (Praxilene) in the treatment of intermittent claudication. Br J Surg 1980;67:347–8.

18. Maass U, Amberger HG, Bohme H, et al. Naftidrofuryl bei arterieller Verschlusskrankheit. Dtsch Med Wochenschr 1984;109:745–50.

19. Zuccarelli F, Marzin L, Landron F. Evaluation of naftidrofuryl for the treatment of vascular leg ulcers. A controlled trial. Sem Hop 1992;68:860–3.

20. Waters KJ, Craxford AD, Chamberlain J. The effect of naftidrofuryl (Praxilene) on intermittent claudication. Br J Surg 1980;67:349–351.

21. Boger RH, Bode-Boger SM, Thiele W, et al. Biochemical evidence for impaired nitric oxide synthesis in patients with peripheral arterial occlusive disease. Circulation 1997;95:2068–74.

22. Girerd XJ, Hirsch AT, Cooke JP, et al. L-arginine augments endothelium-dependent vasodilation in cholesterol-fed rabbits. Circ Res 1990;67:1301–8.

23. Boger RH, Bode-Boger SM, Thiele W, et al. Restoring vascular nitric oxide formation by L-arginine improves the symptoms of intermittent claudication in patients with peripheral arterial occlusive disease. J Am Coll Cardiol 1998;32:1336–44.

24. Creager MA, Gallagher SJ, Girerd XJ, et al. L-arginine improves endothelium-dependent vasodilation in hypercholesterolemic humans. J Clin Invest 1992;90:1248–53.

25. Schellong SM, Boger RH, Burchert W, et al. Dose-related effect of intravenous L-arginine on muscular blood flow of the calf in patients with peripheral vascular disease: a $H_2^{15}O$ positron emission tomography study. Clin Sci (Lond) 1997;93:159–65.

26. Maxwell AJ, Anderson BE, Cooke JP. Nutritional therapy for peripheral arterial disease: a double-blind, placebo-controlled, randomized trial of HeartBar. Vasc Med 2000;5:11–19.

27. Prostanoids for chronic critical leg ischemia. A randomized, controlled, open-label trial with prostaglandin E_1. The ICAI Study Group. Ischemia Cronica degli Arti Inferiori. Ann Intern Med 1999;130:412–21.

28. Scheffler P, de la Hamette D, Gross J, et al. Intensive vascular training in stage IIb of peripheral arterial occlusive disease. The additive effects of intravenous prostaglandin E_1 or intravenous pentoxifylline during training. Circulation 1994;90:818–22.

29. Diehm C, Balzer K, Bisler H, et al. Efficacy of a new prostaglandin E_1 regimen in outpatients with severe intermittent claudication: results of a multicenter placebo-controlled double-blind trial. J Vasc Surg 1997;25:537–44.

30. Mangiafico RA, Messina R, Attina T, et al. Impact of a 4-week treatment with prostaglandin E_1 on health-related quality of life of patients with intermittent claudication. Angiology 2000;51:441–9.

31. Belch JJ, Bell PR, Creissen D, et al. Randomized, double-blind, placebo-controlled study evaluating the efficacy and safety of AS-013, a prostaglandin E_1 prodrug, in patients with intermittent claudication. Circulation 1997;95:2298–302.

32. Loosemore TM, Chalmers TC, Dormandy JA. A meta-analysis of randomized placebo control trials in Fontaine stages III and IV peripheral occlusive arterial disease. Int Angiol 1994;13:133–42.

33. Lievre M, Azoulay S, Lion L, et al. A dose-effect study of beraprost sodium in intermittent claudication. J Cardiovasc Pharmacol 1996;27:788–93.

34. Lievre M, Morand S, Besse B, et al. Oral Beraprost sodium, a prostaglandin I(2) analogue, for intermittent claudication: a double-blind, randomized, multicenter controlled trial. Beraprost et Claudication Intermittente (BERCI) Research Group. Circulation 2000;102:426–31.

35. Mohler ER 3rd, Hiatt WR, Olin JW, et al. Treatment of intermittent claudication with beraprost sodium, an orally active prostaglandin I_2 analogue: a double-blinded, randomized, controlled trial. J Am Coll Cardiol 2003;41:1679–86.

10. PHARMACOTHERAPY FOR GLOBAL CARDIOVASCULAR RISK REDUCTION

Kim A Eagle and Debabrata Mukherjee

Atherothrombosis is the leading cause of death in the United States and contributes to >70% of all deaths (Fig. 10.1).[1] Of the approximately 2 million deaths in the United States in 2001, coronary heart disease or stroke (all-cause) was listed as the primary or contributing cause in approximately 1 391 000 cases.[1] The Centers for Disease Control has postulated that if all forms of atherothrombosis were eliminated, the average life expectancy in the USA would rise by 7 years.[1] Similar trends have been seen in other countries (such as England and Wales, Sweden, Canada, Australia, and Italy) with one-third to over 40% of all deaths due to atherothrombotic disease.[2]

The annual incidence of myocardial infarction (MI) in the USA is 650 000, and the incidence of stroke is about 500 000. The overall prevalence of MI and stroke in the USA is 7.5 million and 4.6 million, respectively.[1] Less is known about the epidemiology of peripheral arterial disease (PAD) than that of MI and stroke. Existing epidemiologic data show wide variations, with reported incidence and prevalence varying with the demographic factors of the specific population being studied (including age, gender, and geographic area)

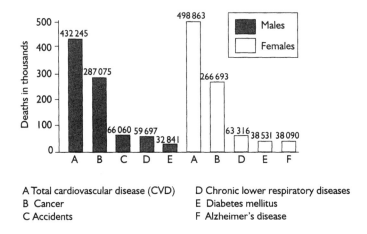

Figure 10.1 *Leading causes of death in the United States in 2001 stratified by gender. (Adapted from AHA.)[1]*

and diagnostic methods employed — questionnaires tend to overestimate the frequency of PAD with symptoms, whereas an objective method of diagnosis, such as a measurement of Doppler systolic ankle pressures, is more accurate.[3] Available epidemiological studies suggest the prevalence of PAD in the population of North America, who are ≥ 55 years old, is about 10.5 million.[4]

Even more worrisome is the fact that the burden of atherothrombosis is growing. It has been estimated that the prevalence of MI and ischemic stroke will rise by approximately one-third from 1997 to 2005.[5] The increase in prevalence of these conditions is growing faster than the elderly population and therefore cannot be entirely explained by changing population demographics. Increased survival after a first event and effective secondary prevention may contribute to this increase in prevalence.

The San Diego Artery Study evaluated the mortality rate from all cardiovascular disease and coronary heart disease (CHD) in a free-living population. Of the 565 subjects examined (average age 66 years), 67 patients (11.9%) were identified as having PAD by noninvasive testing. The patients were then followed prospectively for 10 years. Figure 10.2 shows the Kaplan–Meier survival curves (all-cause mortality) for four groups of patients: normal, asymptomatic, symptomatic, and severely symptomatic.[6] The survival curves demonstrate a poor prognosis for patients with PAD; even asymptomatic patients had sharply reduced survival, compared with normal subjects. The subgroup with severe symptomatic PAD had the worst prognosis: analysis of this group revealed a 15-fold increase in rates of mortality due to cardiovascular disease and CHD. After 10 years, about half

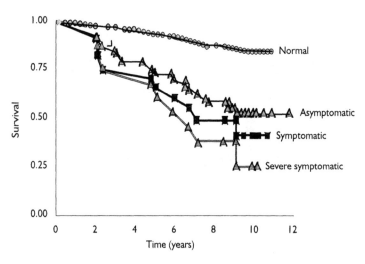

Figure 10.2 *Kaplan–Meier curves for 10-year survival rates of subjects in the San Diego Artery Study stratified by severity of peripheral arterial disease. (Adapted from Criqui et al.)*[6]

of asymptomatic patients had survived, whereas only 25% of severely symptomatic patients had survived.

The overall survival rate for patients with PAD who have intermittent claudication is only 72% at 5 years and approximately 50% at 10 years. These survival rates are much lower than those for age-adjusted controls, for whom the rate is 90% at 5 years. Additional evidence suggests that atherosclerosis in other locations further increases a patient's mortality risk. In fact, 5-year mortality rates in PAD patients are higher than rates in patients with breast cancer or those with Hodgkin's disease (Fig. 10.3). The mortality rate of patients with PAD provides strong evidence that they should receive careful cardiovascular evaluation, and undergo aggressive treatment to manage risk factors such as smoking, hyperlipidemia, hypertension, sedentary lifestyle, obesity, and diabetes.

The previous chapters have discussed the benefits of antiplatelet therapy, beta-blockers, angiotensin-converting enzyme (ACE) inhibitors, and statins in patients with peripheral arterial diseases. In a pilot study, we showed significant incremental beneficial effects of combination evidence-based use of antiplatelet therapy, statins, ACE inhibitors and beta-blockers in patients with PAD, with an improvement in clinical outcomes at just 6 months of follow-up (Table 10.1).[7] For this analysis, an appropriateness algorithm for the use of each of the various secondary prevention strategies was created using evidence-based clinical practice guidelines from the American College of Cardiology (ACC) and the American Heart Association (AHA).[8–10] Class I recommendations from ACC/AHA guidelines were used to develop the

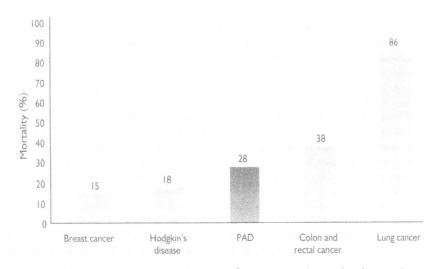

Figure 10.3 *Relative 5-year mortality rates for patients with peripheral arterial disease (PAD) vs other common pathologies. (Adapted from American Cancer Society.)*[13]

131

Table 10.1 Risk-adjusted predictors of clinical outcomes at 6 months in patients undergoing peripheral vascular interventions

	No event (n = 54)	Event (n = 12)	Adjusted odds ratio	95% CI	p-value
Age	65.6 ± 10.3	69.5 ± 12.4	1.05	0.97–1.13	0.25
Diabetes	20.3%	33.4%	3.80	0.65–21.9	0.13
Composite appropriateness	68.3%	48.2%	0.02	0.01–0.44	0.01

Source: adapted from Mukherjee et al.[7]

appropriateness algorithm. Based on this information, patients were considered candidates for lipid-lowering therapy if they had known hyperlipidemia. Hyperlipidemia was defined as meeting any of the following criteria: total cholesterol ≥200 mg/dL, LDL ≥100 mg/dL, triglycerides ≥200 mg/dL, or past/present use of lipid-lowering agents.[11] ACE inhibitors were judged as being indicated for patients with one or more of the following conditions: hypertension, heart failure, diabetes, or a documented ejection fraction (EF) <40%. All patients with PAD were considered candidates for antiplatelet therapy, dietary modification, exercise training, and complete cessation from smoking. Patients with known contraindications to any of these agents, such as ACE inhibitors (intractable cough, angioedema) and beta-blockers (severe heart failure, worsening brochospasm), were excluded from analysis. The percentage of patients on appropriate evidence-based therapy among those considered eligible was then calculated at hospital discharge. For each patient there were four possible recommended drugs: antiplatelet agents, lipid-lowering therapy, ACE inhibitors, and beta-blockers.

In a subsequent report, we demonstrated that the use of combination evidence-based medical therapies was also independently and strongly associated with lower 6-month mortality in patients with acute coronary syndromes (Fig. 10.4). A composite appropriateness score was calculated for each patient on the basis of the number of the drugs used at discharge divided by the number of the drugs indicated, expressed as a percentage. Subsequently, a composite appropriateness level was determined for each patient based on the following algorithm:

0 – none of the indicated medications used (score = 0)
I – 1 medication used if 3 or 4 medications indicated (score = 25 or 33.3)
II – 2 medications used if 3 or 4 medications indicated or 1 medication used if 2 medications indicated (score = 50 or 66.7)

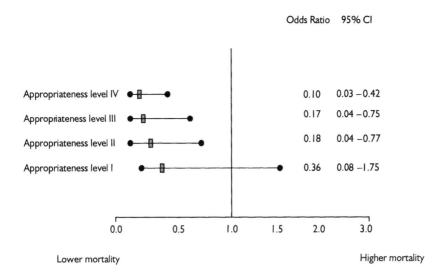

Odds Ratio 95% CI

Appropriateness level IV   0.10   0.03 – 0.42

Appropriateness level III   0.17   0.04 – 0.75

Appropriateness level II   0.18   0.04 – 0.77

Appropriateness level I   0.36   0.08 – 1.75

0.0   0.5   1.0   1.5   2.0   3.0

Lower mortality   Higher mortality

Figure 10.4 *Effect of combined use of evidence-based medical therapies on 6-month mortality in patients with acute coronary syndromes. Composite appropriateness levels (I–IV) are compared with level 0 (non-use of any of the indicated medications) and show a gradient of survival benefit in this cohort. (Adapted from Mukherjee et al.)*[14]

III – 3 medications used if 4 medications indicated (score = 75)
IV – all indicated medications were used (score = 100).

Combination evidence-based medical therapy among eligible patients dramatically lowers 6-month mortality in patients with acute coronary syndromes.

Patients with peripheral vascular diseases represent an important high-risk cohort, where secondary vascular disease prevention is likely to be particularly effective and cost-effective. Clinicians have an opportunity to provide high-quality and appropriate evidence-based care to this high-risk cohort and to seize this opportunity in aggressively treating the underlying atherosclerotic process through lifestyle modifications and effective pharmacological therapies. However, despite strong and unequivocal benefits of these agents, secondary preventive therapies continue to be underutilized, as demonstrated in previous studies. Attention to these 'disease management' opportunities has significant survival advantage in this high-risk cohort and suggests the need for development for quality improvement initiatives geared toward patients with PAD similar to the Guidelines Applied in Practice (GAP)[12] and the Get with the Guidelines programs for patients with coronary disease.

Key points

- Atherothrombosis is the leading cause of death in the United States and contributes to more than 70% of all deaths.
- The global burden of atherothrombosis is growing.
- The overall survival rate for patients with PAD who have intermittent claudication is only 72% at 5 years and approximately 50% at 10 years.
- Combination of evidence-based medical therapies independently and strongly improve clinical outcomes in patients with vascular diseases.
- There is a need for the development for quality improvement initiatives geared toward patients with peripheral vascular diseases to improve and optimize pharmacotherapy.

References

1. AHA. 2004 Heart and Stroke Statistical Update. Dallas, TX, 2004.

2. World Health Organization. www.who.int/whosis/ 2002.

3. Ouriel K. Peripheral arterial disease. Lancet 2001;358:1257–64.

4. Weitz JI, Byrne J, Clagett GP, et al. Diagnosis and treatment of chronic arterial insufficiency of the lower extremities: a critical review. Circulation 1996;94:3026–49.

5. Guillot F, Moulard O. Increasing worldwide prevalence of atherothrombotic manifestations. Circulation 1998;98:1421.

6. Criqui MH, Langer RD, Fronek A, et al. Mortality over a period of 10 years in patients with peripheral arterial disease. N Engl J Med 1992;326:381–6.

7. Mukherjee D, Lingam P, Chetcuti S, et al. Missed opportunities to treat atherosclerosis in patients undergoing peripheral vascular interventions: insights from the University of Michigan Peripheral Vascular Disease Quality Improvement Initiative (PVD-QI2). Circulation 2002;106:1909–12.

8. Braunwald E, Antman EM, Beasley JW, et al. ACC/AHA guideline update for the management of patients with unstable angina and non-ST-segment elevation myocardial infarction – 2002: summary article: a report of the American College of Cardiology/American Heart Association Task Force on Practice Guidelines (Committee on the Management of Patients With Unstable Angina). Circulation 2002;106:1893–900.

9. Cannon CP, Battler A, Brindis RG, et al. American College of Cardiology key data elements and definitions for measuring the clinical management and outcomes of patients with acute coronary syndromes. A report of the American

College of Cardiology Task Force on Clinical Data Standards (Acute Coronary Syndromes Writing Committee). J Am Coll Cardiol 2001;38:2114–30.

10. Gibbons RJ, Abrams J, Chatterjee K, et al. ACC/AHA 2002 guideline update for the management of patients with chronic stable angina – summary article: a report of the American College of Cardiology/American Heart Association Task Force on Practice Guidelines (Committee on the Management of Patients With Chronic Stable Angina). Circulation 2003;107:149–58.

11. Expert Panel on Detection, Evaluation, and Treatment of High Blood Cholesterol in Adults. Executive Summary of The Third Report of The National Cholesterol Education Program (NCEP) Expert Panel on Detection, Evaluation, And Treatment of High Blood Cholesterol In Adults (Adult Treatment Panel III). JAMA 2001;285:2486–97.

12. Mehta RH, Montoye CK, Gallogly M, et al. Improving quality of care for acute myocardial infarction: The Guidelines Applied in Practice (GAP) Initiative. JAMA 2002;287:1269–76.

13. American Cancer Society — Cancer Facts and Figures. 1997.

14. Mukherjee D, Fang J, Chetcuti S, et al. Impact of combination evidence-based medical therapy on mortality in patients with acute coronary syndromes. Circulation 2004;109:745–9.

Venous diseases

11. DEEP VENOUS THROMBOSIS/ PULMONARY EMBOLISM PHARMACOTHERAPY

Douglas E Joseph and John R Bartholomew

Introduction

Traditional pharmacological management for venous thromboembolic disease (VTE) which includes deep vein (venous) thrombosis (DVT) and pulmonary embolism (PE) consists of inpatient anticoagulation with unfractionated heparin (UFH) bridging to an oral anticoagulant (warfarin). In the 1970s and 1980s the low-molecular-weight heparins (LMWHs) were introduced in Europe and have now become readily available in the United States. These preparations, which have the advantages of subcutaneous administration, predictable and stable levels of anticoagulation, lack of a need for laboratory monitoring, and indications for outpatient management of DVT, are rapidly becoming the anticoagulants of choice for treatment of VTE.

In selected patients, the thrombolytic agents (streptokinase, urokinase*, and recombinant tissue plasminogen activator) may be indicated for the management of DVT to restore venous patency or for treatment of the hemodynamically unstable patient or an individual with right ventricular dysfunction with acute pulmonary embolism (PE). More recently Food and Drug Administration (FDA)-approved treatment options for anticoagulation include Fondaparinux, a synthetic pentasaccharide analogue and the direct thrombin inhibitors (DTIs) argatroban, lepirudin, and bivalirudin. Fondaparinux is approved for VTE prevention in patients undergoing total knee or hip replacement, individuals with hip fracture, and inpatient management of VTE. The DTIs currently have no approved indications for the treatment of VTE but are used for one of the most devastating complications of UFH or LMWH, heparin-induced thrombocytopenia (HIT). Argatroban and lepirudin are indicated for the treatment of HIT, whereas argatroban is also approved for the management of HIT in patients undergoing percutaneous coronary intervention (PCI), while bivalirudin is used in non-HIT patients with acute coronary syndromes. Table 11.1 lists the currently available anticoagulants in the United States.

*Urokinase may no longer be available as a thrombolytic agent in the future.

Table 11.1 List of anticoagulants	
Type of anticoagulant	Agents available in the United States
Heparin	Unfractionated heparin
Low-molecular-weight-heparins (LMWHs)	Enoxaparin, dalteparin, tinzaparin
Vitamin K antagonists	Warfarin
Thrombolytic agents	Streptokinase, urokinase, recombinant tissue plasminogen activator complex, reteplase
Synthetic pentasaccharide analogue	Fondaparinux
Direct thrombin inhibitors (DTIs)	Argatroban, bivalirudin, lepirudin

Prevention of venous thromboembolism

VTE is highly prevalent among hospitalized patients and represents a major cause of morbidity and mortality. If unrecognized and untreated, VTE results in death in up to 30% of patients, and is responsible for approximately 200 000 deaths annually in the United States.[1] The mortality rate drops from 30% to as low as 2–8% when VTE is properly recognized and treated.[2,3] VTE can also result in the development of the post-thrombotic syndrome, which is characterized by pain, swelling, and leg ulceration, as well as the disabling symptoms of chronic thromboembolic-induced pulmonary hypertension.

Prevention of VTE is therefore of utmost importance. Unfortunately it is often overlooked and underutilized.[4,5] Thromboprophylaxis should be considered in all hospitalized patients and select outpatients and its use based on an overall assessment of each individual's risk factors. Some of the more common risk factors contributing to the development of VTE are listed in Table 11.2. These are often separated into primary (hereditary) or secondary (acquired) conditions.

Treatment of venous thromboembolism

Goals of therapy include preventing death from PE, avoidance of recurrent VTE, reduction of symptoms and averting the development of the post-thrombotic syndrome and pulmonary hypertension. In 1960, Barritt and Jordan demonstrated that UFH was safe and resulted in reduced death and

Table 11.2 Some of the more common risk factors for venous thromboembolism	
Hereditary or primary risk factors	Acquired or secondary risk factors
• Antithrombin deficiency	• Age
• Protein C deficiency	• Surgery
• Protein S deficiency	• Trauma
• Factor V Leiden	• Prior history of VTE
• Prothrombin gene mutation	• Antiphospholipid antibody syndrome
• Elevated factor VIII levels	• Cancer
• Hyperhomocysteinemia	• Chemotherapy
• Dysfibrinogenemia	• Myocardial infarction, stroke
	• Pregnancy
	• Estrogen therapy
	• Obesity
	• Heparin-induced thrombocytopenia

recurrence of PE when compared to no therapy. Until recently, UFH has been considered the standard of care for the treatment of VTE.[6]

Heparin

UFH is an acidic glycosaminoglycan, with preparations ranging in molecular weight from 5000 to 30 000 Da (mean approximately 15 000 Da). It acts by catalyzing the effect of antithrombin (AT), making it more efficient at combining with and inactivating thrombin (factor IIa). It also inhibits multiple other serine proteases, including factors Xa, IXa, XIa, and XIIa.

Heparin dosing

UFH has a variable anticoagulant dose–response, often leading to difficulty with dosing. A 1993 study compared a weight-based UFH dosing protocol with adjustments made to achieve a target activated partial thromboplastin time (aPTT) of 1.5–2.3 times the control value to more traditional dosing regimens common at that time.[7] The weight-based UFH dosing protocol was found superior to other more traditional methods. Patients in the weight-based group were within the targeted aPTT range within 24 hours of initiating therapy 97% of the time, compared to only 77% of those individuals in the traditional group, and the rate of recurrence was much higher in the latter group. Nomograms are now the accepted method for managing UFH in most institutions. An example of one of the more commonly used nomograms is shown in Table 11.3.

Table 11.3 Weight-based nomogram for heparin[7]

Condition	Procedure
Initial dose	80 units/kg bolus; followed by 18 U/kg/h Check aPTT in 6 hours
aPTT <35 seconds (<1.2 × control)	80 units/kg bolus; then increased by 4 U/kg/h Check aPTT in 6 hours
aPTT, 35–45 seconds (1.2–1.5 × control)	40 units/kg bolus; then increased by 2 U/kg/h Check aPTT in 6 hours
aPTT, 46–70 seconds (1.5–2.3 × control)	No change Check aPTT next day
aPTT, 71–90 seconds (2.3–3 × control)	Decrease infusion rate by 2 U/kg/h Check aPTT next day
aPTT > 90 seconds (>3 × control)	Hold infusion 1 hour; then decrease infusion rate by 3 U/kg/h Check aPTT in 6 hours

aPTT, activated partial thromboplastin time.

Monitoring heparin therapy

UFH is commonly monitored using the aPTT, although the thrombin time (TT), activated clotting time (ACT), or plasma UFH concentrations are also used. The recommended therapeutic range for the aPTT is 1.5–2.5 times each institution's laboratory control value. This should correspond to anti-factor Xa plasma heparin concentrations of 0.3–0.7 IU/mL, measured by an amidolytic assay, or 0.2–0.4 U/mL, as calculated by the protamine titration method.

Earlier clinical trials of the 1970s and 1980s demonstrated that the recurrence of VTE could be minimized by maintaining the aPTT within the therapeutic range, especially during the first 1–3 days following an acute thrombotic event.[8,9] A more recent 1997 double-blind, randomized study re-emphasized this concept, demonstrating VTE recurrence rates of 23.3% in patients who did not attain a therapeutic aPTT level within 24 hours after initiating therapy, compared to a 4–6% rate for those who reached this threshold.[10]

UFH can also be monitored using the plasma UFH levels with therapeutic levels as cited above. These are most useful in individuals with a lupus anticoagulant where the baseline aPTT is elevated, or in patients suspected of heparin resistance.[11] This latter condition is most often encountered in patients with VTE who are acutely ill, in patients with malignancy, inflammatory bowel disease, or during peri- or postpartum periods. Heparin resistance is defined as the requirement for more than 35 000–40 000 U/day of UFH and is the result of elevated factor VIII levels and heparin-binding proteins, including platelet factor 4 (PF4), fibrinogen, and histidine-rich glyocoprotein, which results in a dissociation between the aPTT and plasma heparin values. Heparin resistance is also seen in patients with HIT, antithrombin deficiency (formerly antithrombin III), in patients with large clot burdens (as seen with massive PE), and it has been associated with certain drugs, including aprotinin and nitroglycerin.

The TT is not readily available at most institutions and is not commonly used for monitoring UFH. The ACT is the standard method used to monitor UFH during open-heart or vascular surgery, cardiac catheterization, and percutaneous coronary interventions (PCI), but it is not used for monitoring UFH in patients with VTE.

Duration of therapy with heparin

For many years, the standard approach for treating patients with acute VTE was a 10-day course of UFH, overlapping with warfarin. This approach was questioned in a 1992 study comparing 10 days of UFH, overlapping with warfarin, beginning on the 5th day of hospitalization, to a 5-day overlapping course beginning on day 1 for patients with an acute proximal DVT. Rates of recurrence were infrequent in both groups and the authors concluded that earlier initiation of warfarin could reduce exposure time to UFH (reducing the risk of HIT), potentially reduce bleeding complications, and allow for a more rapid hospital discharge.[12]

Low-molecular-weight-heparins (LMWHs)

The LMWH compounds were introduced in the United States in the 1990s, initially for the prevention of VTE in the orthopedic population. They are now FDA-approved for prophylaxis in both medical and surgical patients as well as for the outpatient treatment of DVT. They are not yet approved for outpatient treatment of acute PE.

LMWHs are created from UFH by enzymatic or chemical degradation to produce mucopolysaccharide species with molecular weights of approximately 5000 Da. LMWHs contain the active pentasaccharide group in lower proportion than standard UFH. Because of its smaller size, LMWH has a reduced ability to catalyze the inhibition of thrombin (factor IIa) but maintains full inhibitory activity against factor Xa.

The LMWHs have a more predictable dose response, longer plasma half-life (allowing for once or twice daily weight-adjusted dosing), are easy to administer, and there is less need for laboratory monitoring. In addition, more than 80% of patients with an acute DVT can be treated without hospitalization.[13] Physicians must recognize that the LMWHs are not interchangeable, however, and each of the available preparations in the United States has its own respective indication and dosing regimen.

Dosing the LMWH preparations

Tables 11.4 and 11.5 list the FDA-approved indications and dosages for the LMWH preparations available in the United States for the treatment or prevention of VTE.

In a meta-analysis of five trials, no significant differences were found with regards to recurrence of VTE or bleeding complications between once- vs twice-daily administration in patients with VTE.[14] All of the currently approved LMWH preparations available in the United States have once-a-day dosing options for treatment or prophylaxis of acute VTE. However, not all preparations are approved for both treatment and prevention.

Box 11.1 lists the minimal elements required for the early discharge or outpatient management of VTE.

Monitoring the LMWH preparations

Laboratory monitoring is generally not recommended except for those patients with renal insufficiency, during pregnancy, and in the obese or pediatric-age

Table 11.4 Dosage of LMWH agents for the treatment of VTE

Agent	Dose
Tinzaparin (Innohep)	175 IU/kg SC q 24 hours
Enoxaparin (Lovenox)	1.5 mg/kg SC q 24 hours or 1 mg/kg SC q 12 hours
Dalteparin* (Fragmin)	200 IU/kg SC q 24 hours or 100 IU/kg SC q 12 hours

Note: Twice-daily (bid) dosing may be preferred in patients with complicated thromboembolic disorders or in patients with high bleeding risk.
*Dalteparin is not approved by the FDA for treatment of VTE in the United States.

Table 11.5 Dosage of LMWH preparations for VTE prophylaxis

Drug	Dose	Indication
Dalteparin (Fragmin)	2500–5000 anti-Xa IU/day	Abdominal surgery, hip replacement surgery and gynecologic and urologic surgery patients
Enoxaparin (Lovenox)	30 mg q 12 h or 40 mg/day	Medical patients, hip, knee or abdominal surgery
Tinzaparin (Innohep)*	3500 anti-Xa IU/day or 50 anti-Xa IU/kg/day	Surgical prophylaxis* Orthopedic surgery* (for orthopedic surgery 75 anti-Xa IU/kg/day)

* Not FDA-approved for this indication.

patient. When required, an anti-factor Xa assay using LMWH as the standard is recommended. This level should be monitored 4 hours after a subcutaneous injection with therapeutic ranges of 0.6–1.0 IU/mL recommended for twice-daily administration and greater than 1.0 for once-a-day administration.

The LMWH preparations are primarily eliminated by the kidneys and have generally been considered contraindicated in patients with renal impairment, defined as a creatinine clearance of 30 mL/min or less.[15] More recently, the manufacturers of enoxaparin sodium (Lovenox) have published dosing guidelines for patients with creatinine clearances under 30 mL/min. These recommendations are shown in Table 11.6. Tinzaparin (Innohep) has been shown to be safe for treating VTE in patients with a creatinine clearance of 20 mL/min or greater, although there are no specific guidelines for it or dalteparin (Fragmin) and warnings are listed in their package inserts.[16]

In general, caution is recommended when using the LMWH agents in patients with renal insufficiency. Nagge et al stress that the LMWHs can accumulate in this patient population and advise that use of anti-Xa LMWH levels for monitoring has not been validated. In addition, not all hospitals have

---

Box 11.1 Inclusion criteria for early discharge or outpatient management of DVT*

- Proximal DVT or symptomatic calf DVT
- Patient should be medically and hemodynamically stable
- Low bleeding risk
- Patient should not have severe renal insufficiency
- Capabilities intact for administration of LMWH and monitoring of warfarin
- Patient understands signs and symptoms of bleeding, recurrent DVT, or PE
- Understanding of what to do in the event of an emergency and follow-up
- Willing and able to be discharged from emergency room or outpatient setting

*Not yet FDA-approved for acute PE.

Table 11.6 Enoxaparin dosing for patients with severe renal impairment (creatinine clearance of <30 mL/min)

Indication	Dosage regimen
DVT prophylaxis	30 mg SC qd
Inpatient acute DVT with or without PE	1 mg/kg SC qd
Outpatient acute DVT without PE	1 mg/kg SC qd

Source: Adapted from the dosing pamphlet provided by Aventis Pharmaceuticals.

access to the anti-Xa LMWH tests.[15] Treatment of VTE with the LMWHs is not recommended in patients on hemodialysis due to a lack of data.

Efficacy of the LMWHs

Two large clinical trials have demonstrated that weight-adjusted subcutaneous LMWH is at least as effective and safe as laboratory-monitored intravenous UFH in hospitalized patients with DVT.[17,18] Randomized trials have also demonstrated the safety and efficacy of outpatient LMWH for individuals with acute DVT when compared to in-hospital UFH patients.[19,20] Similar findings were also reported in two other large trials that demonstrated the efficacy and safety of LMWH in patients with acute PE.[18,21]

More recently, LMWH preparations have been recommended for the treatment of VTE in patients with an underlying cancer as a result of studies demonstrating improved outcome. One recent publication compared the efficacy of LMWH to warfarin in preventing recurrent VTE in this patient population.[22] Individuals with symptomatic DVT or PE were either assigned to receive LMWH once daily for 5–7 days and warfarin for 6 months (international normalized ratio (INR) target 2.5) or LMWH once-daily dosing for 6 months. There were more recurrent thrombotic events in the oral anticoagulant group (probability of recurrence 17%) relative to the LMWH-treated group (9%). There was no statistically significant difference between the groups with regards to bleeding events or mortality rate. Based on this data and other studies, the seventh American College of Chest Physicians (ACCP) conference guidelines on antithrombotic therapy now recommend the use of LMWH for the first 3–6 months of therapy for patients with cancer and VTE.[3]

Complications of heparin and the LMWHs

The most commonly recognized complication of both the UFH and LMWH preparations is bleeding. Unfortunately, another potentially devastating complication, HIT, is often overlooked and under-recognized. HIT is reported to occur in as many as 3–5% of all patients exposed to UFH. It is less common with the LMWH agents. HIT is an immune-mediated syndrome associated with a drop in the platelet count that typically occurs 5–14 days after initial exposure to either UFH or LMWH.[23] It may also occur within hours in patients recently sensitized to either preparation (within the previous 100 days). HIT has more recently been recognized to occur 9–30 days after discontinuation of either UFH or LMWH, and is referred to as 'Delayed HIT'. This form usually occurs after an uneventful exposure to either of these anticoagulants. The patient is often discharged, only to reappear with symptoms of a new venous or arterial thrombosis.

In HIT, the platelet count generally drops below $150\,000/mm^3$, although thrombocytopenia is not essential for the diagnosis. HIT must also be considered when there is a 50% reduction in the platelet count from pre-heparin therapy levels. Laboratory testing is helpful in confirming the diagnosis, and most laboratories have the ability to perform heparin-induced platelet aggregation testing or an enzyme-linked immunosorbent assay (ELISA). Few laboratories perform the serotonin-release assay (SRA), considered by many to be the gold standard for the diagnosis of HIT.

Thrombotic complications include arterial occlusions of the limbs, ischemic strokes, and myocardial infarctions. Venous thromboembolic events (DVT and PE), however, are now recognized to occur more frequently, developing in 4 out of 5 patients. Other less common complications associated with HIT include skin necrosis at the site of injection, anaphylactoid-type reaction with hypertension, tachycardia and respiratory collapse, and adrenal vein thrombosis with hemorrhage. The DTIs are now considered the treatment of choice for HIT and are discussed below.

Bleeding is the major cause of complications for patients receiving either UFH or LMWH. Rates of major bleeding are reported as high as 7% for UFH (fatal bleeding episodes of approximately 2%), whereas major bleeding is around 2% (fatal bleeding 0.8%) with the LMWHs.[24] Levels of serious bleeding are believed related to the intensity of anticoagulation. Other bleeding risk factors include recent surgery or trauma, the concomitant use of aspirin, thrombolytic agents or the glycoprotein IIb/IIIa inhibitors, renal failure, and age over 70 years.

Reversal of UFH can be accomplished rapidly by the administration of protamine sulfate and immediate discontinuation of UFH. It is generally recommended that 1 mg of protamine sulfate be given for every 100 U of UFH administered. It should be given slowly to prevent hypotension or anaphylaxis. Excessive doses of protamine can also cause a paradoxical bleeding disorder. Protamine sulfate does not completely reverse the anticoagulant effects of the LMWH preparations. The recommended dose for reversal is 1 mg for every 1 mg of body weight for enoxaparin and 1 mg for every 100 anti-Xa IU of Fragmin or tinzaparin. It is generally advised that the total dose administered not exceed 50 mg at any one time.

All of the LMWH preparations have package inserts that stress precaution with recent or anticipated neuraxial anesthesia (epidural or spinal anesthesia) due to increased risk of spinal or epidural hematoma and subsequent paralysis.

Other complications of the UFH and LMWH preparations include osteoporosis. This is a result of impaired bone formation and enhanced bone resorption that can lead to spinal fractures. It appears to be less of a risk in individuals who receive the LMWHs.

Warfarin

Warfarin remains the most widely used anticoagulant in the United States and the only oral agent now available. Other previously available oral anticoagulants dicumarol and the indanedione derivative, anisindione, are no longer commercially obtainable. The term warfarin is an acronym for the patent holder, Wisconsin Alumni Research Foundation plus the coumarin-derived suffix.

Warfarin exhibits its anticoagulant effect by inhibiting the vitamin K-dependent γ-carboxylation of coagulation factors II, VII, IX, and X. The antithrombotic properties of warfarin lag behind its anticoagulant effects until a sufficient percent of normal clotting factors have been cleared from the circulation. This coincides with factor activity levels of approximately 20% of normal. Peak effects usually occur 36–72 hours following drug administration, although physicians will occasionally see an initial prolongation of the prothrombin time (PT) after only one or two doses. This reflects reduced factor VII activity (half-life of just 5–7 hours) and does not represent adequate anticoagulation because factors II, IX, and X are not sufficiently decreased. This is the rationale for the ACCP guidelines that recommend overlapping warfarin with UFH or LMWH for at least 4–5 days in patients with acute VTE (to ensure adequate anticoagulation). It is also advised that the INR be ≥2.0 for 2 consecutive days. Failure to follow these recommendations may lead to recurrent VTE.

Dosing warfarin therapy

There is some controversy over the optimal starting dose of warfarin in the treatment of VTE. Two studies have suggested that a 5 mg initial dose leads to less intense anticoagulation, yet still achieves a therapeutic INR within 5 days and does not increase the risk for bleeding.[25,26] Another study, based on outpatients, reported that a 10 mg starting dose achieved a therapeutic INR more rapidly without an increase in bleeding.[27] More recently, McRae and Ginsberg recommended a starting dose of 10 mg in fit outpatients, but advocated using lower doses for hospitalized patients with vitamin K deficiency or liver disease.[28] In general, large loading doses are no longer recommended and a 5 mg dose may be best for the hospitalized patient, while leaving the larger doses of 7.5 and 10 mg to healthy outpatients.

Monitoring the oral anticoagulants

The PT has traditionally been used to monitor warfarin therapy; however, in 1982 the World Health Organization (WHO) recommended physicians use the international normalized ratio. The INR is a method that standardizes PT assays and is the ratio of the patient's PT to a control PT. In 1992, the ACCP antithrombotic therapy guidelines made recommendations based on the INR. The accepted therapeutic INR for patients with VTE is 2–3.

Warfarin can also be monitored using chromogenic assays of the vitamin K-dependent factors II and X. Patients are considered therapeutic when these levels are 20% or lower. This may be especially important in the patient with a lupus anticoagulant where the INR may be slightly prolonged before initiating warfarin. The prothrombin–proconvertin time and Thrombotest have also been used for monitoring oral anticoagulants. Their availability is limited, however, and these tests are unfamiliar to most clinicians.

Duration of therapy with warfarin

Most physicians are unsure how long to treat their patients following an acute VTE event. Studies from the late 1970s and early 1980s demonstrated that individuals with a proximal DVT benefited from 3–6 months of warfarin when compared to only 4–6 weeks of therapy. This time frame reduced the frequency of recurrent VTE from 47% to 2%.[29,30] Several recent publications compared 6 weeks to 6 months of treatment for acute DVT and found recurrence rates significantly lower in the 6-month group.[31,32] Subgroup analysis demonstrated that patients with reversible or temporary risk factors had a lower rate of recurrence and therefore recommended shorter periods of treatment.[31,32]

The recently published 7th edition of the ACCP guidelines recommended dividing the treatment of VTE into five subgroups: these are listed in Table 11.7. Length of treatment ranges from 3 months to indefinite therapy.[3]

Table 11.7 Guidelines for duration of therapy for VTE		
Number of events	Risk factors	Duration of treatment
1st episode	Transient (surgery, trauma)	3 months
1st episode	Cancer	LMWH 3–6 months followed by indefinite treatment (warfarin) until cancer resolved
1st episode	Idiopathic	6–12 months, consider indefinite treatment
1st episode	Hereditary risk factors or other markers identified	6–12 months EXCEPTIONS: Indefinite treatment recommended for patients with the antiphospholipid antibody syndrome, homozygous for factor V Leiden or 2 or more thrombophilic conditions, then indefinite treatment indicated
2 or more episodes objectively documented	None identified	Indefinite treatment

Source: adapted from 2004 ACCP Antithrombotic Therapy Consensus Guidelines.

Intensity of anticoagulation

In 2003, the *New England Journal of Medicine* published two papers that dealt with intensity of therapy for long-term management of patients with idiopathic VTE.[33,34] The Prevention of Recurrent Venous Thromboembolism (PREVENT) trial treated patients with an idiopathic VTE for a median of 6.5 months with conventional therapy and then assigned them to placebo or low-intensity warfarin with a target INR of 1.5–2.0. There was a 48% reduction in the composite end point of recurrent VTE, major hemorrhage, and death in the low-intensity group, with a reduction in the risk of recurrent VTE of 76–81%.[33]

In contrast, the Extended Low-Intensity Anticoagulation for Thromboembolism (ELATE) trial compared low-intensity warfarin (INR 1.5–1.9) to a conventional target range INR of between 2.0 and 3.0. This study found the incidence of recurrent VTE significantly greater in the low-intensity warfarin group (16 of 369 had recurrent VTE) compared with those assigned to the conventional-intensity warfarin therapy group (6 of 369).[34]

The most recent ACCP guidelines do not recommend lower-intensity anticoagulation for long-term treatment of patients with VTE.[3]

Complications of warfarin therapy

On a yearly basis major bleeding with long-term warfarin anticoagulation occurs in 1–3% of all patients, while minor bleeding occurs in approximately 6–10%.[35] The risk of bleeding appears to increase with the length and intensity of therapy as well as in those individuals with a history of stroke, gastrointestinal bleeding, and age over 65 years.[24]

In the setting of life-threatening bleeding, prompt reversal of warfarin therapy can be attained by the use of intravenous vitamin K, fresh frozen plasma, prothrombin complex concentrates, or recombinant factor VIIa. The recommended dose for vitamin K is 10 mg given slowly intravenously, while fresh frozen plasma should be given at 15 mL/kg.[35] Frequent monitoring of the INR should be performed and patients may require additional doses of these agents.

Although either prothrombin complex concentrate or recombinant factor VIIa may be necessary in a life-threatening situation due to warfarin overdose, most physicians are unfamiliar with their use and it may be advisable to obtain the recommendations of consultants more familiar with these agents.

Warfarin-induced skin necrosis (WISN) is an unusual but potentially devastating complication of therapy in patients with VTE. It generally occurs between days 3 and 5 of therapy and is often associated with the administration of larger initial loading doses of an oral anticoagulant. WISN has been linked to hereditary deficiencies of protein C, and protein S, antithrombin, resistance to activated protein C, and the antiphospholipid antibody syndrome. It is the result of a transient hypercoagulable state due to a rapid decrease in the levels of protein C and factor VII. Patients initially develop an erythematous, flushed, area on the skin that progresses to petechial hemorrhages and eventual skin infarction. These lesions are very painful and most frequently involve the breasts, thighs, or buttocks. Women appear more likely to develop WISN than men. Immediate discontinuation and reversal of warfarin is recommended using vitamin K and fresh frozen plasma. Alternative anticoagulants are usually necessary and UFH or LMWH should be administered unless the patient has HIT. The combination of HIT and WISN has recently been recognized in a number of patients while receiving both UFH and warfarin in the management of VTE. In most cases, HIT was not recognized and the patients receiving warfarin or an equivalent oral anticoagulant had a supratherapeutic INR. Venous limb gangrene occurred in many of these patients. This syndrome should be preventable by not initiating warfarin in patients with HIT until the patient is improving clinically, using smaller doses initially and waiting until the platelet count has recovered to at least $100\,000/mm^3$ and preferably to $150\,000/mm^3$.[36]

Other well-known complications of warfarin include fetal embryopathy, occurring between the 6th to 12th week of gestation, and the atheromatous embolization syndrome. It is imperative that physicians inform their patients of the potential harm that can occur if they become pregnant while taking warfarin. Atheromatous embolization is characterized by purple toes and is generally seen following percutaneous invasive or surgical procedures.

Thrombolytic therapy for VTE

There are four thrombolytic agents currently available in the United States and streptokinase (SK), urokinase (UK), and recombinant tissue plasminogen activator (rt-PA) are currently approved by the FDA for the management of VTE.

The use of thrombolytic agents is often controversial and must be highly individualized. Thrombolytic therapy for acute DVT is generally reserved for younger individuals with an iliofemoral or axillary-subclavian DVT. In addition, patients with phlegmasia cerulea dolens (venous gangrene), without bleeding risk, or individuals with occluded central venous catheters, needing continued intravenous access, might be candidates for this therapy. In patients with an acute DVT, it is believed that resolution of the clot will result in restoration of venous patency and avoid the complications of the post-thrombotic syndrome.

Although most patients with acute PE are hemodynamically stable and can be managed effectively with UFH, a small percentage (less than 5–7%) will present with hemodynamic compromise. These patients usually have a massive PE and present with hypotension and circulatory collapse requiring more aggressive therapy. In this setting, most clinicians favor the use of thrombolytic therapy over pulmonary embolectomy, assuming no contraindications exist for its use. Thrombolysis accelerates resolution of the PE, improving right

151

ventricular function, pulmonary perfusion, and the hemodynamic status of the patient. Unfortunately, no large clinical trials to date have demonstrated a reduction in mortality utilizing these agents.

A number of physicians also recommend thrombolytic therapy for hemodynamically stable patients with echocardiographic findings of right ventricular dysfunction. In this subgroup of patients, the goal of therapy is rapid reversal of right-sided dysfunction, with the potential for leading to a reduction in death and recurrent pulmonary emboli. According to Goldhaber et al, these patients have 'impending hemodynamic instability' and represent up to 40–50% of all normotensive patients presenting with acute PE.[37] Reportedly, recurrence and death rate for PE is higher in patients with right ventricular dysfunction, despite their normotensive presentation.

In the Management Strategy and Prognosis of Pulmonary Embolism Registry (MAPPET) the relationship between thrombolysis treatment and heperin and prognosis of hemodynamically stable patients with major PE was examined.[38] The 30-day mortality was significantly lower in patients who received thrombolytic agents, and patients who underwent early thrombolytic therapy also had a reduction in recurrent PE. Major bleeding was increased with thrombolysis.[38] This study had limitations, however, because it was a registry.

More recently, MAPPET-3 compared the effects of thrombolysis to UFH on the prognosis of patients with acute submassive PE who had right ventricular strain.[39] The results suggested superiority of thrombolytic therapy with respect to clinical deterioration; however, they again did not demonstrate a decrease in recurrent PE or in hospital mortality.

Most studies demonstrate a favorable outcome for patients who present with an acute PE, are hemodynamically stable, and are treated with UFH or LMWH. Although thrombolytic therapy results in more rapid resolution of PE initially, this still has not yet conclusively translated into a reduction in mortality or reduction in the rate of recurrent PEs. In patients with smaller emboli that do not produce hemodynamic compromise, thrombolytic therapy is not yet warranted. In the patient with a massive PE, thrombolytic therapy is recommended but not based solely on the echocardiographic findings. Prospective studies are needed to determine if patients with right ventricular dysfunction will benefit from this more aggressive approach.

Dosing guidelines
Recommended dosing guidelines for the thrombolytic agents are found in Table 11.8. Contraindications, both relative and absolute, are listed in Table 11.9.

Bleeding is the major risk for patients receiving thrombolytic therapy, with the major concern being intracranial hemorrhage, which is reported to occur in between 0.5% and 2% of all patients.[3,35] Immediate discontinuation of the thrombolytic agent is recommended if serious bleeding develops.

Table 11.8 Thrombolytic therapy for acute PE or DVT

Agent	FDA approval for PE or DVT	Dosing protocols
Streptokinase*	PE and DVT	250 000 U over 30 min followed by 100 000 U/h for 24 hours
Urokinase*	PE	4400 U/kg over 10 min followed by 4400 U/kg for 12 hours
rt-PA†	PE	100 mg over 2 hours
Reteplase†	None	2 separate boluses of 10 U approximately 30 min apart

* Not recommended to use heparin concurrently with SK or UK.
† Heparin is optional for rt-PA and reteplase.

Table 11.9 Contraindications for thrombolytic therapy

Absolute	Relative
Recent major trauma or surgery (within 10 days)	Prolonged cardiopulmonary resuscitation
Recent cerebrovascular accident (within 2 months) or intracranial malignancy	Pregnancy
Bleeding diathesis or active internal bleeding	Diabetic proliferative retinopathy
Recent intracranial or intraspinal surgery (within 2 months)	Severe hypertension (systolic > 180 mmHg and diastolic > 110 mmHg)

Cryoprecipitate, which contains high levels of fibrinogen, should be given: also consider the addition of an antifibrinolytic agent such as ε-aminocaproic acid (Amicar).

Newer anticoagulants

A number of new anticoagulants have been developed during the past decade as alternatives to UFH and LMWH therapy in the treatment of VTE. These include a selective inhibitor of factor Xa and the direct thrombin inhibitors.

Fondaparinux

Fondaparinux (Arixtra) is a parenteral synthetically prepared pentasaccharide analogue that has been approved for the prevention and treatment of VTE. It is a selective inhibitor of factor Xa that is dependent on antithrombin. It has advantages of rapid absorption, 100% bioavailability, single fixed dose, and a half-life of 17 hours, allowing for once-daily administration. Fondaparinux does not affect the aPTT or ACT. It is renally excreted, and therefore precaution must be used in patients with renal insufficiency. Fondaparinux does not appear to cross-react with heparin-induced antibodies, and monitoring the platelet count may not be necessary.

Dosing recommendations for VTE prophylaxis are 2.5 mg daily, whereas dosing for the treatment of VTE ranges from 5 mg for patients under 50 kg, to 7.5 mg for those individuals weighing between 50 and 100 kg to 7.5 mg for those over 100 kg.

The FDA approved fondaparinux in December 2001 for DVT prophylaxis in patients undergoing hip fracture, hip replacement, and knee replacement surgery based on studies demonstrating fewer VTE events when compared to the LMWH enoxaparin. There was no significant difference in major bleeding episodes, although the doses for enoxaparin differed in several of the studies.[40,41]

Fondaparinux has also been compared with enoxaparin for the initial treatment of DVT and UFH for the initial treatment of PE. In the MATISSE-DVT trial and MATISSE-PE trial, rates of symptomatic, recurrent VTE and major bleeding were not different.[42,43] Fondaparinux is now approved for inpatient treatment of both of these conditions.

There have been no reported cases of HIT or cross-reactivity of heparin platelet factor 4 antibodies with fondaparinux; therefore, its use for prophylaxis of VTE in orthopedic surgery patients and treatment of acute VTE in patients with a history of HIT may be ideal.

There is no specific antidote for fondaparinux, although recent recommendations suggest that recombinant factor VIIa may be of help in emergency situations.[42]

Direct thrombin inhibitors

Argatroban, lepirudin, bivalirudin: Three DTIs have been approved for use in the United States. Argatroban and the hirudin derivative lepirudin (Refludan) have been approved for treatment of HIT. Argatroban also has indications for prophylaxis and use in patients with HIT who require PCI. Both agents have been compared to historical controls in patients with HIT and demonstrated favorable outcomes.[44] Argatroban has a short half-life (39–51 min) and the advantage that no dose adjustment is required for patients with renal dysfunction. Dosing adjustments are necessary for patients with liver disease.

Lepirudin has a half-life of 1.3 hours and requires dosing adjustments for patients with renal disease because of its mechanism for excretion, but no adjustment for patients with liver impairment. Antihirudin antibodies have been reported to develop in up to 40% or more of patients that are re-exposed to lepirudin. Both agents can be monitored using the aPTT.

Bivalirudin (Angiomax) is approved for patients with unstable angina and the acute coronary syndrome. It is not used for the acute treatment of VTE, nor is it approved for patients with HIT.

Ximelagatran: Ximelagatran is an oral DTI. It is a prodrug of melagatran that blocks thrombin's interaction with its substrates.[45] It has a half-life of 3–5 hours and therefore must be administered twice per day. The kidneys eliminate most of the drug. Monitoring is not necessary because it produces a predictable anticoagulant response, although it does prolong the aPTT and INR. The Thrombin Inhibitors in Venous Thromboembolism (THRIVE) treatment study demonstrated that ximelagatran was as effective as conventional anticoagulation in the prevention of recurrent VTE.[45] It had been predicted that this agent would soon be available in the United States to compete with warfarin for long-term anticoagulation in patients with VTE. Unfortunately, one if its side effects (elevation of liver enzymes in as many as 5–10% of patients) may have led to a recent decision by the FDA not to approve this drug.

Alternative treatment options for acute VTE: inferior vena cava filters

Inferior Vena Cava (IVC) filters protect against fatal PE and as many as 40 000 are placed every year in the United States.[46] Patients with a contraindication to anticoagulation, individuals with recurrent VTE despite adequate anticoagulation, patients who are undergoing pulmonary embolectomy, and those with a complication of anticoagulation are absolute candidates for these devices. The absolute and relative indications for the placement of IVC filters are found in Table 11.10.

Table 11.10 Indications for IVC filters

Absolute	Relative
Contraindication to anticoagulation	Massive pulmonary embolism
Failure of adequate anticoagulation	Primary prophylaxis
Complication of anticoagulation	Free-floating thrombi
Patients undergoing surgical pulmonary embolectomy	Chronic cardiac or pulmonary insufficiency

A large trial examining the effectiveness of IVC filters enrolled 400 patients with proximal DVT and assigned patients to receive standard anticoagulation or an IVC filter. During the first 12 days, significantly fewer patients in the IVC filter group suffered PE. After 2 years there were no significant differences in survival or symptomatic PE. However, patients who received an IVC filter had a 21% rate of recurrence of a DVT, compared with 12% of those who did not receive a filter.[46] Based on this study it is usually advised that patients be anticoagulated following IVC filter placement, once it becomes safe to do so.

IVC filters also migrate, penetrate organs, and occasionally form clots above the filter. It is speculated that the introduction of temporary IVC filters would minimize and/or eliminate those problems. Indications for temporary IVC filters may eventually include surgical or trauma patients, the young or pregnant patient, and patients who require thrombolysis for an actue DVT when there is concern for embolization.

A summary of management strategies for the treatment of VTE is given in Figure 11.1

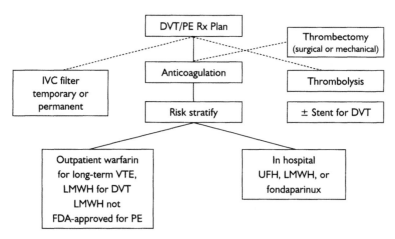

Figure 11.1 Summary of management strategies for the treatment of VTE

Key points
Prevention of VTE
- VTE prevention is important but is often overlooked and underutilized.
- Preventive measures include mechanical agents (aggressive mobilization after surgery, elastic graduated compression stockings, intermittent pneumatic compression) and pharmacotherapy agents including warfarin UFH, LMWH, and fondaparinux.

Treatment of VTE
- Goals of therapy include preventing death from PE, preventing thrombus propagation, reducing symptoms, minimizing recurrence, avoiding the development of the post-thrombotic syndrome and chronic pulmonary hypertension.
- Treatment with an immediate-acting anticoagulant (UFH, LMWH, and, more recently, fondaparinux) followed by early initiation of a vitamin K antagonist is standard therapy.
- Use of the thrombolytic agents may be indicated in patients with iliofemoral DVT or massive PE.
- An IVC filter is generally indicated in patients in whom anticoagulation is contraindicated.

Heparin
- Heparin remains an important anticoagulant in the management of VTE because of physician familiarity, its effectiveness and low cost.
- The target aPTT of 1.5–2.5 times the control should be attained as quickly as possible to prevent recurrent VTE.
- Heparin can lead to devastating complications, including HIT.

Low-Molecular-Weight-Heparin
- The development of LMWH has allowed outpatient treatment of DVT due to a more predictable dose response, longer plasma half-life, once- or twice-daily weight-adjusted dosing, and less need for laboratory monitoring.
- LMWHs are not yet FDA-approved for the outpatient management of acute PE.
- LMWH is eliminated by the kidney; thus caution should be given to its use in patients with renal impairment.

Warfarin
- Warfarin is currently the only oral anticoagulant available for long-term management of VTE in the United States.
- Peak effect occurs 36–72 hours following drug administration and initial prolongation of the PT generally reflects reduced factor VII activity. This does not represent adequate anticoagulation because the intrinsic clotting pathway remains active until factors II, IX, and X are sufficiently reduced (about 5 days).
- UFH and warfarin must be overlapped at least 4–5 days in patients with acute thrombosis.
- Duration of therapy with warfarin varies from 3 to 6 months for a temporary or situational VTE to indefinite for recurrent or idiopathic events.

- Warfarin-induced skin necrosis is a rare complication of the oral anticoagulants and usually develops 3–5 days after initiating this agent.

Thrombolytic therapy for VTE

- Use of thrombolytic agents in VTE is controversial and must be highly individualized.
- Patients with acute PE who are hemodynamically unstable or younger individuals who have an iliofemoral DVT and are at low risk for bleeding are the most appropriate candidates.

New anticoagulant agents

- Newer agents include the selective inhibitors of factor Xa and the DTIs.
- Fondaparinux is now approved for the prevention and inpatient treatment of VTE and has advantages of once-daily administration.
- The DTIs have indications for the treatment of HIT, and there are two agents available (argatroban and lepirudin). Caution should be used with argatroban in patients with liver disease and lepirudin in patients with renal impairment.
- Ximelagatran was not approved by the FDA in the United States due to liver toxicity.

IVC filters

- IVC filters are indicated in patients with a contraindication to anticoagulation, a failure of adequate anticoagulation, a complication of anticoagulation, or if the patient is to undergo pulmonary embolectomy.
- The temporary filters may replace permanent filters in the near future.

References

1. Horlander KT, Mannino DM, Leeper KV. Pulmonary embolism mortality in the United States, 1979–1998: an analysis using multiple-cause mortality data. Arch Intern Med 2003;163(14):1711–17.

2. Douketis JD, Kearon C, Bates S, Duku EK, Ginsberg JS. Risk of fatal pulmonary embolism in patients with treated venous thromboembolism. JAMA 1998; 279(6):458–62.

3. Buller HR, Agnelli G, Hull RD, et al. Antithrombotic therapy for venous thromboembolic disease. Chest 2004;126(3):401–28.

4. Anderson FA Jr, Wheeler HB, Goldberg RJ, Hosmer DW, Forcier A. Physician practices in the prevention of venous thromboembolism. Ann Intern Med 1991;115(8):591–5.

5. Bratzler DW, Raskob GE, Murray CK, Bumpus LJ, Piatt DS. Underuse of venous thromboembolism prophylaxis for general surgery patients: physician practices in the community hospital setting. Arch Intern Med 1998;158(17):1909–12.

6. Barritt DW, Jordan SC. Anticoagulant drugs in the treatment of pulmonary embolism. A controlled trial. Lancet 1960;1:1309–12.

7. Raschke RA, Reilly BM, Guidry JR, Fontana JR, Srinivas S. The weight-based heparin dosing nomogram compared with a 'standard care' nomogram. A randomized controlled trial. Ann Intern Med 1993;119(9):874–81.

8. Basu D, Gallus A, Hirsh J, Cade J. A prospective study of the value of monitoring heparin treatment with the activated partial thromboplastin time. N Engl J Med 1972;287(7):324–7.

9. Hull RD, Raskob GE, Hirsh J, et al. Continuous intravenous heparin compared with intermittent subcutaneous heparin in the initial treatment of proximal-vein thrombosis. N Engl J Med 1986;315(18):1109–114.

10. Hull RD, Raskob GE, Brant RF, Pineo GF, Valentine KA. Relation between the time to achieve the lower limit of the APTT therapeutic range and recurrent venous thromboembolism during heparin treatment for deep vein thrombosis. Arch Intern Med 1997;157(22):2562–8.

11. Hirsh J, Warkentin TE, Shaughnessy SG, et al. Heparin and low-molecular-weight heparin: mechanisms of action, pharmacokinetics, dosing, monitoring, efficacy, and safety. Chest 2001;119:64S–94S.

12. Hull RD, Raskob GE, Rosenbloom D, et al. Heparin for 5 days as compared with 10 days in the initial treatment of proximal venous thrombosis. N Engl J Med 1990;322(18):1260–4.

13. Wells Philip S, Kovacs MJ, Bormanis J, et al. Expanding eligibility for outpatient treatment of deep venous thrombosis and pulmonary embolism with low-molecular-weight heparin: a comparison of patient self-injection with homecare injection. Arch Intern Med 1998;158:1809–12.

14. Couturaud F, Julian JA, Kearon C. Low molecular weight heparin administered once versus twice daily in patients with venous thromboembolism: a meta-analysis. Thromb Haemost 2001;86(4):980–4.

15. Nagge J, Crowther M, Hirsh J. Is impaired renal function a contraindication to the use of low-molecular-weight heparin? Arch Intern Med 2002;162(22):2605–9.

16. Siguret V, Pautas E, Fevrier M, et al. Elderly patients treated with tinzaparin (Innohep) administered once daily (175 anti-Xa IU/kg): anti-Xa and anti-IIa activities over 10 days. Thromb Haemost 2000;84(5):800–4.

159

17. Hull RD, Raskob GE, Pineo GF, et al. Subcutaneous low-molecular-weight heparin compared with continuous intravenous heparin in the treatment of proximal-vein thrombosis. N Engl J Med 1992;26(15):975–82.

18. Simonneau G, Sors H, Charbonnier B, et al. A comparison of low-molecular-weight heparin with unfractionated heparin for acute pulmonary embolism. The THESEE Study Group. Tinzaparine ou Heparine Standard: Evaluations dans l'Embolie Pulmonaire. N Engl J Med 1997;337(10):663–9.

19. Levine M, Gent M, Hirsh J, et al. A comparison of low-molecular-weight heparin administered primarily at home with unfractionated heparin administered in the hospital for proximal deep-vein thrombosis. N Engl J Med 1996;334(11):677–81.

20. Koopman MM, Prandoni P, Piovella F, et al. Treatment of venous thrombosis with intravenous unfractionated heparin administered in the hospital as compared with subcutaneous low-molecular-weight heparin administered at home. The Tasman Study Group. N Engl J Med 1996;334(11):682–7.

21. Low-molecular-weight heparin in the treatment of patients with venous thromboembolism. The Columbus Investigators. N Engl J Med 1997;337(10):657–62.

22. Lee AY, Levine MN, Baker RI, et al. Low-molecular-weight heparin versus a coumarin for the prevention of recurrent venous thromboembolism in patients with cancer. N Engl J Med 2003;349(2):146–53.

23. Warkentin TE, Levine MN, Hirsh J, et al. Heparin-induced thrombocytopenia in patients treated with low-molecular-weight heparin or unfractionated heparin. N Engl J Med 1995;332(20):1330–5.

24. Levine MN, Raskob G, Landefeld S, Kearon C. Hemorrhagic complications of anticoagulant treatment. Chest 2001;119:108S–121S.

25. Harrison L, Johnston M, Massicotte MP, et al. Comparison of 5 mg and 10 mg loading doses in initiation of warfarin therapy. Ann Intern Med 1997;126:133–6.

26. Crowther MA, Ginsberg JB, Kearon C, et al. A randomized trial comparing 5-mg and 10-mg warfarin loading doses. Arch Intern Med 1999;159:46–8.

27. Kovacs MJ, Rodger M, Anderson DR, et al. Comparison of 10-mg and 5-mg warfarin initiation nomograms together with low-molecular-weight heparin for outpatient treatment of acute venous thromboembolism. A randomized, double-blind, controlled trial. Ann Intern Med 2003;138:714–19.

28. McRae SJ, Ginsberg JS. Initial treatment of venous thromboembolism. Circulation 2004;110(suppl I):I-3–I-9.

29. Hull R, Delmore T, Genton E, et al. Warfarin sodium versus low-dose heparin in the long-term treatment of venous thrombosis. N Engl J Med 1979;301(16):855–8.

30. Hull R, Delmore T, Carter C, et al. Adjusted subcutaneous heparin versus warfarin sodium in the long-term treatment of venous thrombosis. N Engl J Med 1982;306(4):189–94.

31. Schulman S, Rhedin AS, Lindmarker P, et al. A comparison of six weeks with six months of oral anticoagulant therapy after a first episode of venous thromboembolism. Duration of Anticoagulation Trial Study Group. N Engl J Med 1995;32(25):1661–5.

32. Hirsh J, Bates SM. Clinical trials that have influenced the treatment of venous thromboembolism: a historical perspective. Ann Intern Med 2001;134(5):409–17.

33. Ridker PM, Goldhaber SZ, Danielson E, et al. Long-term, low-intensity warfarin therapy for the prevention of recurrent venous thromboembolism. N Engl J Med 2003;348:1425–34.

34. Kearon C, Ginsberg JS, Kovacs MJ, et al. Comparison of low-intensity warfarin therapy with conventional-intensity warfarin therapy for long-term prevention of recurrent venous thromboembolism. N Engl J Med 2003;349:631–9.

35. Warkentin TE. Reversing anticoagulants both old and new. Can J Anesth 2002;49:S11-S25.

36. Srinivasan AF, Rice L, Bartholomew JR, et al. Warfarin-induced skin necrosis and venous limb gangrene in the setting of heparin-induced thrombocytopenia. Arch Intern Med 2004;164:66–70.

37. Goldhaber SZ, Haire WD, Feldstein ML, et al. Alteplase versus heparin in acute pulmonary embolism: randomized trial assessing right-ventricular function and pulmonary perfusion. Lancet 1993;341:507–11.

38. Konstantinides S, Geibel A, Olschewski M, et al. Association between thrombolytic treatment and the prognosis of hemodynamically stable patients with major pulmonary embolism: results of a multicenter registry. Circulation 1997;96(3):882–8.

39. Konstantinides S, Geibel A, Heusel G, Heinrich F, Kasper W. Heparin plus alteplase compared with heparin alone in patients with submassive pulmonary embolism. N Engl J Med 2002;347:1143–50.

40. Eriksson BI, Bauer KA, Lassen MR, Turpie AG. Fondaparinux compared with enoxaparin for the prevention of venous thromboembolism after hip-fracture surgery. N Engl J Med 2001;345(18):1298–304.

41. Bauer KA, Eriksson BI, Lassen MR, Turpie AG. Fondaparinux compared with enoxaparin for the prevention of venous thromboembolism after elective major knee surgery. N Engl J Med 2001;345(18):1305–10.

42. Buller HR, Davidson BL, Decousus H, et al. Fondaparinux or enoxaparin for the initial treatment of symptomatic deep venous thrombosis. Ann Intern Med 2004;140:867–73.

43. The Matisse Investigators. Subcutaneous fondaparinux versus intravenous unfractionated heparin in the initial treatment of pulmonary embolism. N Engl J Med 2003;49:1695–702.

44. Hirsh J, Heddle N, Kelton J. Treatment of heparin-induced thrombocytopenia: a critical review. Arch Intern Med 2004;361:361–9.

45. Schulman S, Wahlander K, Lundstrom T, Clason SB, Eriksson H. Secondary prevention of venous thromboembolism with the oral direct thrombin inhibitor ximelagatran. N Engl J Med 2003;349(18):1713–21.

46. Decousus H, Leizorovicz A, Parent F, et al. A clinical trial of vena caval filters in the prevention of pulmonary embolism in patients with proximal deep-vein thrombosis. Prevention du Risqué d'Embolie Pulmonaire par Interruption Cave Study Group. N Engl J Med 1998;338(7):409–15.

12. COMPRESSION THERAPY AND INJECTION SCLEROTHERAPY FOR VENOUS DISEASE

Rupal Dumasia and John Pfeifer

Introduction

Chronic venous insufficiency (CVI) is a problem that affects approximately 5 million people in the United States.[1] Of these people, 400 000–500 000 have or will develop a venous leg ulcer. The prevalence of venous disease is higher in industrialized countries than in other countries.[2] It is more common in women than in men and in older than in younger people. The Tecumseh Community Health Study showed that 72% of women aged 60–69 have CVI, but 1% of men aged 20–29 have CVI.[3] The prevalence of CVI is expected to rise with the aging population in this country.

CVI encompasses a spectrum of clinical manifestations which include edema, hyperpigmentation, venous stasis dermatitis, chronic cellulitis, cutaneous infection, lipodermatosclerosis, ulceration, and malignant degeneration.[2] Venous ulceration is a chronic and recurrent problem. According to studies based on patient recall, 50% of ulcers are present for 7–9 months, up to one third are present for more than 5 years, and 67–75% of patients have recurring ulcers.[1] Given the scope of the problem, as well as its chronic and recurrent nature, prevention and treatment are of paramount importance. The treatment can be divided into mechanical, pharmacological, and surgical modalities. This chapter will focus on the rationale and appropriate use of mechanical therapies, including medical elastic compression stockings, and will provide an overview of sclerotherapy.

History of compression

Compression bandages have been used since the times of the ancient Egyptians. Fabrizio d'Aquapendente introduced leggings and lace-up stockings made of dog leather in the 16th century for the treatment of various leg conditions. Theden, one of Frederick the Great's surgeons, was instrumental in reintroducing compression bandages to the German-speaking countries in the 18th century.

Modern medical compression bandages were not truly developed until the proper materials were developed. Rubber was elastic enough to exert pressure and stretched enough to allow patients to wear the leggings. The problem was that the leggings were prone to overheating, leading to skin damage, and they quickly became brittle. In 1839, Charles Goodyear discovered that if rubber was heated, its elasticity and durability would remain but its negative characteristics would be eliminated. The term 'vulcanization', referring to this process, was coined by Thomas Hancock.

Despite the rapid advances in technology, compression stockings did not gain the widespread approval of physicians until the early 20th century. After several symposia, it was decided that stockings should be divided into standard compression classes. In 1970, the Hohenstein Research Institute developed uniform testing standards for compression stockings. Thus, centuries of technological advances and cooperation between physicians and engineers have led to the modern medical elastic stocking.[4]

Pathophysiology of venous insufficiency

To understand the rationale for the use of medical elastic compression stockings, one needs to understand normal venous physiology and venous pathophysiology. In order for venous return from the leg to reach the right heart, it must overcome gravity, waxing and waning thoracoabdominal pressures, and sometimes elevated right atrial pressure (right heart failure). This requires a complex series of properly functioning valves and pumps. In addition, the circuit must be patent.

The calf muscle pump is often thought of as a peripheral heart.[2] When the muscles of the calf contract, they compress the pumping chamber in the calf. The pumping chamber of the calf is the intricate network of unusually distensible veins (sinuses) of the gastrocnemius and soleus muscles. These sinuses empty into the tibial veins as well as the popliteal vein. The compression of the pumping chamber pushes blood up towards the heart. When the muscles relax, the sinuses of the calf expand and allow blood to enter from the superficial collecting system of the leg.

The calf muscle pump depends on normally functioning one-way valves to prevent regurgitation of venous blood. Venous valves are bicuspid and are found every few centimeters in the deep and superficial veins of the leg below the common femoral vein. They are normally able to withstand pressures of up to 3 atmospheres (atm). After calf muscle contraction, the blood from the lower extremity is pumped out of the leg by the calf muscle action on the chamber. As the calf muscle chamber dilates after contraction, the venous sinuses which constitute the chamber have a lower pressure than the superficial leg veins (a gradient of 100–110 mmHg). This results in flow from the superficial veins to the chamber of the calf muscle. Arterial inflow is the other source of blood that fills the chamber. After a period of prolonged standing, the venous system is full, and the valves are open. The hydrostatic pressure is then equal to the height of a column of blood from head to toe. This increase in hydrostatic pressure triggers an urge to move the lower extremity and activate the calf muscle pump. The next contraction of the calf muscles pumps the blood from within the chamber into the venous outflow tract.

The two major causes of venous insufficiency are impaired outflow and retrograde inflow. The problem may lie in the deep or superficial venous system. The etiology can be related to failure of the calf muscle pump, venous obstruction, valvular incompetence, or a combination of these. Calf muscle failure may be due to muscle wasting, neuromuscular disease, or prolonged standing. In this case, the immediate postambulatory venous pressure is as high as the pressure after prolonged standing. Less venous blood is pumped into the circulation. The arterial inflow is compromised, because arterial blood enters a higher pressure system. This contributes to ischemia and ulceration.

Significant obstruction (thrombotic or nonthrombotic) of the deep venous system may lead to inability of the distal deep veins to empty. In this case, the calf muscle pump is working properly, but the outflow tract is partially or completely obstructed.

The most common cause of symptomatic venous disease is valve failure. For a variety of reasons, including inflammation, cytokine release, thrombosis, and congenital lesions, the valves may be incompetent and permit reflux from the deep to superficial or from proximal to distal veins. Moreover, venous distention may lead to failure of a normal valve to close, because the leaflets can no longer form a tight seal. This is analogous to regurgitation of cardiac valves due to annular dilatation. Thus, some evidence indicates that reflux is probably due to a weakening of vein walls and subsequent venous dilatation, resulting in incompetence of the valve. This is an instance in which external compression is helpful in restoring valve competence.[2,5]

Deep vein valve incompetence leads to a rapid increase in venous filling and pressure after standing. This leads to the same sequelae as calf muscle pump failure. The same problem can affect valves of the perforator veins. In this situation, the high pressure generated by the normal calf muscle pump is transmitted to the superficial veins through the incompetent perforator valves. The thin-walled superficial veins dilate in response to this high pressure and form varicosities. Valvular incompetence can occasionally be limited to the superficial veins. This may occur as a result of local trauma, superficial phlebitis, hormonal influence (pregnancy), or congenital lesions. This does not lead to hemodynamic sequelae but does cause local symptoms. Valve incompetence can also occur at the junction of the greater saphenous vein with the common femoral vein or the lesser saphenous vein with the popliteal vein. These are the largest of the perforator veins. This leads to constantly elevated venous pressure in the superficial system and may result in local skin damage by edema, inflammation, or ulceration.[2]

Physiology of compression

Compression therapy is based upon physical and chemical principles. The physics of compression is far better understood than the biochemical effects. Edema can be thought of as fluid that has extravasated from the vasculature into the interstitial space. The fluid, however, is not inert and does lead to adverse biochemical changes in the surrounding tissue. Compression can counteract some of these changes. For example, it does improve the ability of tissue to participate in fibrinolysis.[6]

The distinction between compression bandages and stockings must be made prior to discussing physical principles. Compression bandages are made from a variety of materials with differing elastic properties. Stockings are made from relatively elastic materials. The less elastic the stocking, the more difficult it is to put on, and the more anti-edema effect it has. The elasticity of a stocking can be quantified using the elasticity coefficient (EC).[7] EC is defined as the ratio of the change in pressure at the B level (ankle) to the change in circumference (D_p/D_o). Figure 12.1 illustrates the concept that stockings can

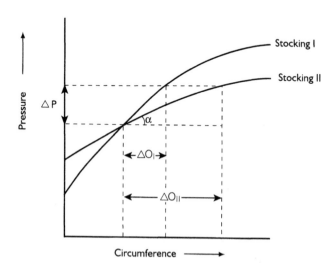

Figure 12.1 Pressure–circumference relationship. The elasticity coefficient is tan α ($\Delta P/\Delta O$). Stocking I has a higher elasticity coefficient than stocking II.

have different elastic properties. The other distinction between bandages and stockings is that bandaging technique can be modified to change the elastic properties. Stockings have fixed elasticity properties until they are worn out.[6] In general, bandages are used to treat leg ulcers, phlebitis, and other dermatologic problems related to venous stasis until they are under control. Stockings are used as adjunctive and maintenance therapy in this situation. Many patients may need to wear pressure-gradient stockings on a lifelong basis.

Stockings and bandages exert pressure along the axis of the limb. They do not directly push blood upwards against gravity. Their main function is to provide extra support to the affected veins so that the intrinsic mechanisms can operate more effectively. Dilated veins are constricted to allow the valves to function properly. The narrowed veins cause blood to travel faster. This also promotes decreased thrombosis. Also, the extra support decreases the distensibility of the veins and promotes forward movement of blood. Moreover, since edema fluid is incompressible, the pressure exerted from the outside promotes re-entry into the venous side of the capillary loop.[6]

The way that stockings exert pressure on the limb must be understood in the context of the phases of walking. The *working phase* of walking is the phase in which the foot is plantarflexed. During this phase, the calf expands and stretches the stocking laterally, and the ankle extends and stretches it longitudinally. The counterpressure exerted by the stocking on the leg against the pressure by the leg on the stocking is the *working pressure*.[6] This is quantified by the quotient of the work of the calf and the extension of the stocking. The more the stocking yields, the less the effective working pressure.

The *resting phase* of walking is the phase in which the calf relaxes and the foot eases back into neutral position. During this phase, the tension that is stored in the stocking recoils against the leg. The greater the elastic tension and the state of stretch of the stocking, the greater will be the *resting pressure* of the stocking. This can be quantified as the product of the elastic tension of the stocking and the state of stretch of the stocking.[6]

The working pressure and resting pressure have different effects on the venous system. A compression device such as a bandage or a stocking with a very high EC does not yield in response to the work of the calf. The pressure during the working phase of walking will, therefore, be transmitted to the deep veins of the leg. This prevents retrograde flow of blood in the deep veins. Bandages or stiff stockings are used in cases of incompetence of valves in the deep venous system. They do not exert much pressure during the relaxation phase.

In contrast to bandages, stockings with a low EC are highly distensible and yield to the work of the calf. They do not exert much pressure during the working phase. They do, however, recoil during the resting phase. This prevents reflux of blood from the deep to the superficial venous system.

These concepts have been tested in clinical studies. Zajkowski et al used air

167

plethysmography (APG) to study venous hemodynamics in 11 patients with CVI.[8] APG uses a calibrated cuff to encircle the leg and determine changes in leg volume. Venous volume (VV) is the amount of blood in the leg, and venous filling time (VFT) 90 is the time it takes for the leg to fill up with 90% of the VV upon standing. These are measures of reflux. The ejection volume (EV) is the amount of blood ejected with a single tiptoe motion, and the ejection fraction (EF) is the fraction of the total blood volume of the leg which is ejected with 1 tiptoe motion (EV/VV). These are measures of calf muscle pump function. In this study, there was a trend toward improvement in measures of reflux with stockings (knee-high, 30–40 mmHg). Stockings provided no benefit in measures of calf muscle pump function.

Jones et al studied the physiological effects of compression in normal controls, patients with superficial varicose veins, and patients with post-phlebitic limbs.[9] They used stockings with 20 mmHg, 30–40 mmHg, and 40–50 mmHg compression at the ankle. Post-phlebitic limbs were found to have improved EV and EF with 40–50 mmHg compression at the ankle. This suggests that patients with deep venous insufficiency have improved calf muscle pump function with high levels of compression because of high working pressure exerted by these stockings.

van Geest et al studied the effect of EC on capillary filtration rate (CFR) and edema in patients with known CVI.[10] In this study, patients were randomized to stockings with low EC and 30 mmHg compression, high EC and 30 mmHg compression, and low EC and 34.5 mmHg compression. APG was used to measure EC and calculate CFR. CFR was significantly higher in the group not wearing stockings than in the other groups. CFR was higher in the low-EC, 30 mmHg compression group compared with the other two groups. There was no difference in CFR between the high-EC group and the low-EC, high-compression group. This suggests that stockings with lesser elasticity are better for edema prevention than more elastic stockings.

Indications for compression

The indications for compression stockings become rather obvious after understanding the pathophysiology of venous insufficiency. CVI is generally a process that progresses slowly and often goes undetected until it becomes severe. Compression stockings of varying classes can be useful for a broad spectrum of patients with CVI.

Prevention in healthy patients
One indication for compression is for the prevention of the late skin damage of CVI. For healthy patients, the best way to prevent damage to leg veins is

movement. This is not always possible, particularly for those with sedentary or standing occupations. Weiss and Duffy studied the effect of ready-to-wear (RTW) lightweight gradient compression stockings (8–15 mmHg and 15–20 mmHg) on subjective symptoms of 19 flight attendants over a 4-week period.[11] RTW hosiery was effective in improving discomfort, swelling, fatigue, and aching. There was no difference between 8–15 mmHg stockings and 15–20 mmHg stockings.

Jonker et al conducted a similar study to test the effect of support stockings on diurnal volume change (DVC) in 118 healthy subjects.[12] This study tested stockings exerting an average pressure of 18 mmHg (stocking Y), 14 mmHg (stocking X), and 6 mmHg (stocking Z). The latter was used as a control stocking. Stockings X and Y led to less diurnal volume increase than stocking Z. This relationship was true for both men and women. There was an improvement in subjective complaints of 'tired/heavy legs' and 'swollen ankles/feet' with stockings X and Y. There was no difference in subjective complaints between stockings X and Y.

Prevention in pregnancy

Pregnancy is another indication for the use of compression as preventive therapy. Pregnant women are prone to varicose veins for a number of reasons, including increased blood volume, hormonally mediated dilation of veins, and uterine compression of the inferior vena cava. These changes usually return to baseline after pregnancy. The varicose veins may become permanent after several pregnancies. Patients who are susceptible should be fitted with 20–30 mmHg graduated compression stockings or a pregnancy pantyhose to wear throughout pregnancy. This will reduce long-term varicose vein development. Patients with a history of varicose veins should use 30–40 mmHg stockings. If this is uncomfortable, calf-length 20–30 mmHg stockings can be worn over 20–30 mmHg pantyhose.[2]

Post-sclerotherapy compression

Compression should also be used as an adjunct to vein sclerotherapy. Adjunctive compression decreases local thrombophlebitis after the procedure and prevents the occurrence of new varicose veins at 1 year. Compression hose also prevents reflux through incompetent perforators, which may flush out the sclerosing agent at the time of injection. Also, compression decreases the amount of local thrombus formation, and as a result, decreases the likelihood of recanalization. The decrease in thrombus formation also protects against post-sclerosis pigmentation.

Although deep venous thrombosis is related to injection technique, the incidence of superficial thrombophlebitis after sclerotherapy can be decreased if compression is instituted. This may be due to decreased extension of thrombus through perforator veins or decreased direct endothelial injury. Finally, compression leads to direct apposition of treated vein walls and, therefore, a greater treatment effect with a lower concentration of sclerosing agent. This has been borne out in a clinical study in which 20–30 mmHg of compression after sclerotherapy led to improved results.[2,13] The authors believe that the majority of deep vein thromboses during sclerotherapy relate to the technique of injection.

The duration of compression after sclerotherapy is a matter of debate. There is evidence that even a few days of compression immediately after sclerotherapy can provide a benefit over no compression at all. One study suggested that 1 week of compression is better than 3 days, and 3 weeks is even better.[13] One approach would be to use uninterrupted compression for the first 3 days, followed by 2–3 weeks of compression interrupted only for showers.[2]

The authors use compression continuously for 3 days and 2 nights followed by 2 weeks of daytime use. This protocol is repeated each time sclerotherapy is carried out. Long-term use of stockings to prevent recurrence is recommended and decreases the recurrence rate by 70%.

Contraindications to compression

Although a wide range of patients with venous disease benefit from compression stockings, there are some groups of patients who cannot tolerate them. This may be for anatomic or physiologic reasons. Patients with severe edema, weeping stasis dermatitis, or new venous ulcers benefit more from bandages, rest, and elevation in the acute phase. Once the edema has improved and open lesions are controlled, compression stockings should be used. In addition, the cause of edema must be carefully determined. Edema due to heart failure should not be treated with compression. Forcing fluid back into the circulation may lead to pulmonary edema. If patients with compensated heart failure develop venous insufficiency, compression can be used.

Arterial insufficiency is the other major contraindication to the use of compression. It is important to check arterial pulses before and after application of compression bandages. Even the presence of pulses does not guarantee adequate tissue perfusion. Intracompartmental pressures can be as high as 80 mmHg with normal arterial pulses. If pulses are absent, ankle–brachial indexes should be calculated prior to compression: 20–30 mmHg hose are usually safe with early arterial occlusive disease. Ischemic skin lesions such as ulcers or gangrene preclude the use of pressure gradient stockings in such patients. Often the first sign of excessive compression is pain/discomfort. It is very important to instruct patients to remove stockings immediately if they experience pain. Some authors recommend wearing two pairs of stockings for additive compression; however, it is important to remove the outer stocking during sleep. In the supine position, there may be tissue hypoperfusion, which is not present while standing.

Other potential problems with stockings may be related to skin irritation or inability to put on the stockings. This may be a problem in the elderly. As mentioned, additive compression may be achieved by using two stockings with less compression. Each stocking individually may be easier to wear.

Manufacture, quality and care of compression stockings

Although compression stockings have theoretical benefits, the translation of these benefits into clinical improvements depends on the proper manufacture, testing, fitting, and care of stockings. The pressure characteristics of compression stockings are fixed at the time of production and are only altered when the stocking is worn out. The stockings can be made by the flat-knitting or circular-knitting technique.

Flat-knitting technique

The modern flat-knitting machine has two opposing rows of needles. The fabric is woven when a carriage moves back and forth across the rows of needles. Thin yarns allow for finer knits. The flat material is closed to form a stocking by a seam in the back. The advantage of the flat-knitting technique is that the stockings can be made in any size or shape. Moreover, the stockings can be made to exert high pressures. The durability is also an advantage. The disadvantage is that the knit is coarser than circular knitting, and there is a seam. This may make the flat-knit stocking less aesthetically appealing.[14] An example of this type of stocking commercially available includes the 'vascular seamed garment' (Beiesdorf-Jobst, Inc., Charlotte, NC).

Circular-knitting technique

The circular-knitting machine has needles arranged in a circle. There are more stitches per inch than in the flat-knitting technique. This allows for a much finer knit. The cylinders spin past the knitting points. The knitted stocking is removed from the cylinder by an air blower or a mechanical roller device. All the stitch functions, including the pattern and stitch length, are controlled by an electronic control system. The number of needles and the diameter or the cylinder cannot be changed, but the cylinder can be lowered or raised. Thus, the stocking knit can be made tighter or looser.

In addition to the stitches made by the needles, there are elastic yarns that run in a circumferential direction. The tension of these yarns can be programmed up to a maximum value by computer. Because of the constraints, circular knitting can be used to make stockings for legs whose thigh girth is 2.5–3 times the ankle girth.[14] In general, circular–knit stockings are more attractive and less expensive than flat-knit stockings, but have limited shapes, sizes, and compression. An example of a commercially available circular-knit stocking is the 'seamless soft stocking' (Beiersdorf-Jobst, Inc., Charlotte, NC). All stockings made by Sigvaris (Peachtree City, GA) are circular-knit stockings.

Standard and made-to-measure stockings

The decision to use standard or made-to-measure stockings depends on the dimensions of the patient's leg. Most major manufacturers adhere to the GZG (Quality Seal Association for Medical Compression Stockings) reference table of sizes shown in Figure 12.2.[2] Standard stockings can be circular-knitted or flat-knitted. Standard circular-knitted stockings come in six sizes (I–VI), based on leg circumference measurements at six locations. Standard flat-knitted stockings come in 11 sizes (4–14), based on heel dimensions.

Made-to-measure stockings are produced individually for patients who do not fit into standard sizes. Historically, made-to-measure stockings were flat-knitted, but now circular-knitted stockings can be made-to-measure.

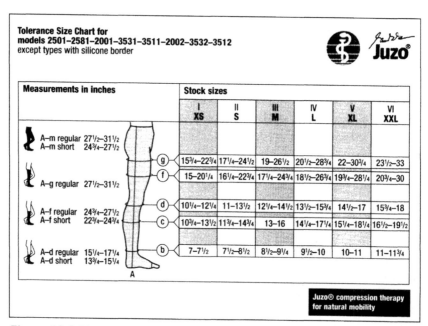

Figure 12.2 Measurement points and size chart for compression stockings.

Quality requirements

The GZG (Quality Seal Association for Medical Compression Stockings) was founded in 1955 by several German compression hosiery manufacturers in order to develop guidelines for the manufacture of quality stockings. These guidelines were developed in conjunction with the German Working Group on Phlebology. Today, the major manufacturers produce stockings which conform to these guidelines and bear the seal of the GZG.

There are several medical requirements that must be fulfilled in order to conform to the guidelines:

- the stockings are distinct from cosmetic stockings
- they must be produced in uniform compression classes
- they must have medically correct pressure gradients
- they must conform to a uniform measurement table
- the heel must be closed.

The quality requirements specify that the stockings must have longitudinal and transverse stretch properties, and seams must be durable and without a raised welt. The exact materials that are permissible are also specified. The amount of compression must fit into a compression class. There are four compression classes, based on the amount of pressure exerted at the 'B' point: this is at the ankle. Table 12.1 shows the compression classes. There must also be continuous pressure drop from the heel to the thigh. This is shown in Figure 12.3.[14]

Care of medical compression stockings

With proper care, stockings should have a life span of 4–6 months. Sweat, soaps, creams, and daily stretch and relaxation contribute to the gradual loss of compression. Toenails should be trimmed to avoid tearing the threads. Rubber gloves should be used when putting the stockings on to prevent tears

Table 12.1 Classes of compression stockings and indications[10]

Compression class	Pressure at B-level (mmHg)	Indications
I	15–21	Thrombosis prophylaxis
II	23–32	Mild/moderate edema, mild CVI, post-sclerotherapy, pregnancy
III	34–46	Severe edema, severe CVI, post-thrombotic syndrome, lymphedema
IV	>48	Severe lymphedema, lipedema

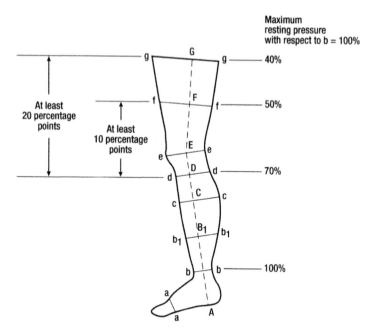

Figure 12.3 *Pressure gradient of medical elastic compression stockings and positions of measurement points.*

from fingernails. Creams, ointments, oils, or solvents should be avoided. Most stockings can be machine washed on a gentle cycle with warm water. Gentle detergents without bleach should be used. Stockings should be air-dried on a flat rack. They should not be hang-dried or machine-dried.

Prescribing medical compression stockings

The effectiveness of the stocking depends not only on the design and patient compliance but also on the prescription of the appropriate stocking. Many physicians either do not include sufficient information on the prescription or they include incorrect information. A complete prescription should include the number of stockings, the compression class, length, type of attachment, standard or made-to-measure, and any additional explanations.[15]

The number of stockings to prescribe is largely a financial decision. It may depend on the stipulations of the insurance company. Ideally, the patient should have two pairs to allow for alternation between washing.

Compression class
The compression classes shown in Table 12.1 are based on the pressure exerted at the ankle. The indication for compression should dictate which compression

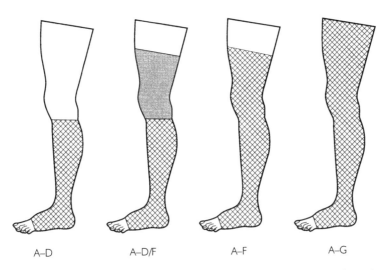

| A–D | A–D/F | A–F | A–G |

Figure 12.4 Stocking lengths: knee-length stockings = A–D; knee-length stockings = A–D/F (with tricot top); mid-thigh-length stockings = A–F; thigh-length stockings = A–G.

class is chosen. Class I stockings are used for thrombosis prophylaxis without edema. Class II should be used in patients with mild-to-moderate edema, post-sclerotherapy, marked varicose veins, and post-sclerotherapy. Class III should be used for post-thrombotic edema and as adjunctive therapy for ulcers. Class IV should be used for severe edema and for lymphedema.

Stockings of higher compression class are more difficult to put on. One way to solve this problem is to prescribe two stockings of a lower compression class to be worn on top of each other. The compression will be roughly additive, and each stocking will be easier to put on. This may be of particular importance in elderly patients.

Measurement and length
The GZG reference table is shown in Figure 12.2. This table is used to determine the appropriate size of standard circular-knit stockings. The circumference of the leg is measured at six places, although fitting is primarily based on the ankle circumference. This is because the stocking exerts 100% of its rated pressure at the ankle. Simplified measurements include the circumference at the ankle, calf, and thigh. The lengths are measured from the heel to popliteal fossa for knee-high stockings and from heel to gluteal fold for thigh-high stockings and pantyhose. The stockings come in three lengths: knee-length (A–D), mid-thigh (A–F), and thigh-length (A–G). Figure 12.4 is a schematic diagram of the different stocking lengths.

Mid-thigh or thigh-length stockings are indicated for varices of the knee and thigh or after sclerosing therapy of these regions. Also, if the circumference of the widest region of the calf (C) does not significantly exceed the circumference of the leg at the knee (D), then a thigh-length stocking may be required.

Attachment

Proper attachment of the stocking to the leg is important. For example, knee-length stockings may creep down if the top of the stocking is not significantly smaller in circumference than the calf. In this case, a thigh extension for attachment to a girdle or garter belt may be helpful (A–D stocking with a D–F extension).[15] This may also be helpful for patients with a significant amount of adipose tissue hanging over the top edge of a knee-high stocking. Thus, it is important to consider attachment of the stocking to the leg. We prefer the alternative of using pantyhose to attachments for poorly fitting stockings.

Standard vs made-to-measure stockings

Made-to-measure stockings are more expensive than standard stockings; however, the consequences of a poorly fitting stocking are even more costly. There are several situations in which made-to-measure stockings are appropriate. Some examples of size-related situations include very large patients and patients with partial amputations/deformities that result in length discrepancies between legs; there are patients in whom the relationship of leg length and girth deviate from the size chart; patients may be intolerant to various materials; and patients may have specific pressure requirements.

In general, the circumference of the leg should be smaller than the corresponding measurement of the stocking. A discrepancy of one stocking size can be tolerated at level D or higher as long as the leg is smaller than the stocking. If the leg is alternately smaller and larger than the corresponding measurements in the size chart, then a made-to-measure stocking is indicated. The fit of the stocking is more important for higher compression classes than lower, because small changes in circumference lead to large changes in pressure.[15]

Pelottes and Laplace's Law

According to Laplace's Law, the pressure of the stocking is directly proportional to the tension and inversely proportional to the radius. No pressure is exerted on flat surfaces, because the radius is infinite. Tight corners are subjected to high pressures because of the small radius. This has important implications on the prescription of stockings. The pressure for which a stocking is rated is based on the assumption that the ankle is a perfectly round structure with a constant radius. This is true for the model on which the stockings are tested (Hohenstein leg), but not for human legs. Veraart et al performed a study to determine the pressure exerted on the medial aspect at the B area by class II compression stockings.[16] According to the CEN classification system, class II stockings should exert a pressure of 25–35 mmHg. Using an electropneumatic system, the pre-

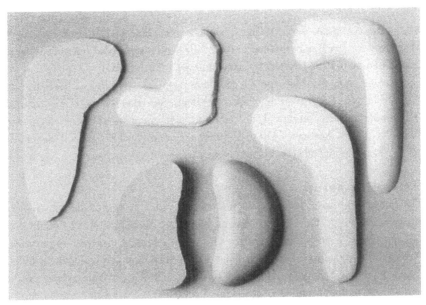

Figure 12.5 *Different kinds of pelottes that can be built into the stocking in order to increase pressure on flat surfaces.*

tibial zone was subject to a pressure of 33.9 mmHg, and the medial site was subject to a pressure of 18.3 mmHg. The pressure on the medial site was found to be below the rated pressure. The problem with this is that 80% of venous ulcers occur on the medial aspect of the leg.

One way to resolve this issue is to use higher-pressure stockings. Another way is to use a pelotte, which is a foam pad with a rounded surface. Figure 12.5 shows examples of pelottes. These may be separate or built into the stocking.

Sclerotherapy and sclerosing agents

Principles, indications, and contraindications

Injection sclerotherapy is a technique in which a small volume of an irritant agent (sclerosant) is injected into a vein in order to obliterate the lumen.[17] The goal is to irreversibly obliterate the lumen by damaging the endothelium and allowing the exposed media to heal by fibrosis. Thrombosis is ideally kept to a minimum, because thrombosed veins can recanalize.[2] This is most commonly performed on incompetent varicose veins or telangiectasias.

Classic teaching is that sclerotherapy is acceptable if there is competence of the saphenofemoral junction, but has a very high recurrence rate in cases of saphenofemoral incompetence.[18] The rationale is that surgery closes the

177

'floodgate' of the junction, but sclerotherapy cannot do this adequately. This is a matter of debate with the use of duplex ultrasound-guided sclerotherapy.[19] The authors ligate incompetent greater or lesser saphenous veins and large incompetent perforators before sclerotherapy is undertaken.

Certain patients are poor candidates for sclerotherapy because of comorbidities. Patients at high risk for deep vein thrombosis (DVT) should not undergo sclerotherapy. This includes patients with a limited ability to ambulate, prior history of DVT or pulmonary embolus (PE), family history of DVT/PE, known hypercoagulable state, or recent pregnancy.[2]

Sclerosing agents

The ideal sclerosant would have no systemic toxicity and would be rapidly inactivated with dilution upon entering the deep venous system. It would take a long time to work, and therefore, be more effective in vessels with stasis. It would not produce local reactions if it extravasates. It would be painless upon injection. There is no perfect solution, but the available agents can be used in a way that simulates these ideal properties.[2] Sclerosing agents can be classified into hypertonic agents, detergent solutions, and corrosive agents. Many are not FDA-approved for sclerotherapy.

Hypertonic agents

Hypertonic saline with or without dextrose works by dehydrating cells and also denaturing cell surface proteins. The advantages of this agent are that it gets diluted rapidly and causes less hyperpigmentation than other solutions. The disadvantages are that it is nonselective and can cause scarring and ulcers if it extravasates. The nonselective nature means that it may affect local nerves and cause a painful response. In addition to hypertonic saline, dextrose and hypertonic saline (10% sodium chloride, 25% dextrose, and a small quantity of phenethyl alcohol) is another hypertonic agent. This agent is produced in Canada under the trade name Sclerodex. It is not approved by the FDA for commercial sale in the United States.

Detergent solutions

These agents are long-chain fatty alcohol molecules that individually have no sclerosing activity. When the concentration of these molecules reaches the critical micellar concentration (CMC), additional molecules form amphiphilic bilayers called micelles. The micelles disrupt the endothelial surface proteins. They do not cause intravascular coagulation. The changes, as observed by a light microscope, take several hours to occur. The extent of damage can be altered by the concentration and the amount of time the solution is in contact with the vessel.

Examples of detergent solutions include polidocanol (POL), sodium tetradecyl sulfate (STS), ethanolamine oleate, and sodium morrhuate. POL is always painless and is effective at low concentrations, but can cause urticaria at the injection site or painless skin necrosis if injected into an arteriole. It is not yet approved for use in the United States. STS has the advantage of being painless when intravascular but painful with extravasation. Skin necrosis and post-sclerosis pigmentation can occur. Sodium morrhuate is a mixture of salts of fatty acids from cod liver oil. It is used for treatment of esophageal varices. It is not recommended for use in treating varicose veins because of a high rate of anaphylaxis and a potential for extensive skin necrosis. Ethanolamine oleate is not recommended for treatment of peripheral varicosities for similar reasons.

Corrosive agents

Corrosive agents comprise a diverse group of agents which poisons the cell surface proteins. The members of this group range from alcohols to heavy metals. They are consumed in the process of acting on the cells; therefore, they are not effective at distant sites. Strong corrosives can affect the full thickness of the vessel wall and are well suited to treat large vessels.

Polyiodinated iodine is the strongest of all available corrosives. It is converted to iodide (non-reactive) when diluted by blood, so it causes a localized reaction. It does cause painful extravasation necrosis. It is highly thrombogenic. Its main use is to sclerose the saphenofemoral and saphenopopliteal junction. Chromated glycerin is a weak agent that does not cause extravasation necrosis. The disadvantage is that it is often too weak. Its main use is for telangiectasias. It is not used in varicose veins. It is often called the 'beginner's sclerosant.'[2]

Key points

- Compression stockings can be used to prevent or treat incompetence of the deep or superficial venous system depending on the elasticity coefficient and compression class.
- Compression therapy is contraindicated in patients with advanced arterial insufficiency and decompensated heart failure.
- Compression stockings must fit properly in order to have a beneficial effect and to prevent complications.
- A complete prescription for compression stockings includes measurements, length, size, and compression class.
- Sclerotherapy is most commonly used to treat telangiectasias and superficial varicosities.
- Compression therapy is required as an adjunct to sclerotherapy.
- Sclerosing agents can be hypertonic, detergent, or corrosive.

References

1. Alguire PC, Mathes BM. Chronic venous insufficiency and venous ulceration. J Gen Intern Med 1997;12:374–83.

2. Weiss RA, Feied CF, Weiss MA. Vein diagnosis and treatment: a comprehensive approach. New York: McGraw-Hill; 2001.

3. Coon WW, Willis PW, Keller JB. Venous thromboembolism and other venous diseases in the Tecumseh Community Health Study. Circulation 1973;48:839–46.

4. Hohlbaum GG. The history of medical compression hosiery. In: GZG (Quality Seal Association for Medical Compression Stockings), ed. The medical compression stocking. New York: Schattauer;1989:107–13.

5. Beebe-Dimmer JL, Pfeifer JR, Engle JS, Schottenfeld D. The epidemiology of chronic venous insufficiency and varicose veins. Arch Epidemiol (in Press).

6. Schmitz R. The importance of medical compression stockings. In: GZG (Quality Seal Association for Medical Compression Stockings), ed. The medical compression stocking, New York: Schattauer;1989:1–38.

7. Neumann HA. Compression therapy with medical elastic stockings for venous diseases. Dermatol Surg 1998;24:765–70.

8. Zajkowski PJ, Proctor MC, Wakefield TW, et al. Compression stockings and venous function. Arch Surg 2002;137:1064–8.

9. Jones NA, Webb PJ, Rees RI, Kakkar VV. A physiological study of elastic compression stockings in venous disorders of the leg. Br J Surg 1980;67:569–72.

10. van Geest AJ, Veraart JC, Nelemans P, Neumann HA. The effect of elastic compression stockings with different slope values. Dermatol Surg 2000;26:244–7.

11. Weiss RA, Duffy D. Clinical benefits of lightweight compression: reduction of venous related symptoms by ready-to-wear lightweight gradient compression hosiery. Dermatol Surg 1999;25:701–4.

12. Jonker MJ, deBoer EM, Ader HJ, Bezemer PD. The edema-protective effect of Lycra support stockings. Dermatology 2001;203:294–8.

13. Weiss RA, Sadick NS, Goldman MP, Weiss MA. Post-sclerotherapy compression: controlled comparative study of duration of compression and its effect on clinical outcome. Dermatol Surg 1999;25:105–8.

14. Weber R. Manufacture, characteristics, testing, and care of medical compression hosiery. In: GZG (Quality Seal Association for Medical Compression Stockings), ed. The medical compression stocking. New York: Schattauer;1989:79–105.

15. Hohlbaum GG. The prescribing of medical compression stockings. In: GZG (Quality Seal Association for Medical Compression Stockings), ed. The medical compression stocking. New York: Schattauer;1989:48–58.

16. Veraart JC, Pronk G, Neumann HA. Pressure differences of elastic compression stockings at the ankle region. Dermatol Surg 1997;23:935–9.

17. Tisi PV, Beverly CA. Injection sclerotherapy for varicose veins (Cochrane Review). In: The Cochrane Library, Issue 1. Chichester, UK: John Wiley and Sons;2004.

18. Hobbs JT. Compression sclerotherapy in venous insufficiency. Acta Chir Scand Suppl 1988;544:75–80.

19. Kanter A, Thibault P. Saphenofemoral incompetence treated by ultrasound-guided sclerotherapy. Dermatol Surg 1996;22:648–52.

INDEX

- Page references to figures and tables are shown in **bold**
- Clinical trials and studies have been indexed as their abbreviated forms